P9-DBX-925

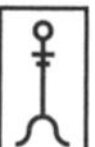

The Complete Guide to Getting a Swimmer's Body

# GET WET, GET FIT

MEGAN QUANN JENDRICK

AND NATHAN JENDRICK

A FIRESIDE BOOK
PUBLISHED BY SIMON & SCHUSTER
New York London Toronto Sydney

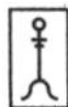

Fireside
A Division of Simon & Schuster, Inc.
1230 Avenue of the Americas
New York, NY 10020

Copyright © 2008 by Megan Jendrick and Nathan Jendrick

All rights reserved, including the right to reproduce
this book or portions thereof in any form whatsoever.
For information address Fireside Subsidiary Rights Department,
1230 Avenue of the Americas, New York, NY 10020

First Fireside trade paperback edition January 2008

FIRESIDE and colophon are registered trademarks of Simon & Schuster, Inc.

For information about special discounts for bulk purchases,
please contact Simon & Schuster Special Sales at 1-800-456-6798
or business@simonandschuster.com

Designed by Jan Pisciotta

Manufactured in the United States of America

10 9 8 7 6 5 4 3 2 1

Library of Congress Cataloging-in-Publication Data

Jendrick, Megan Quann.
Get wet, get fit : the complete guide to a swimmer's body / Megan Quann Jendrick and Nathan Jendrick.
p. cm.
Includes index.
I. Swimming—Training. 2. Physical fitness. I. Jendrick, Nathan. II. Title.
GV837.7.J46 2008
797.2'1—dc22 2007016022

ISBN-13: 978-1-4165-4078-6
ISBN-10: 1-4165-4078-4

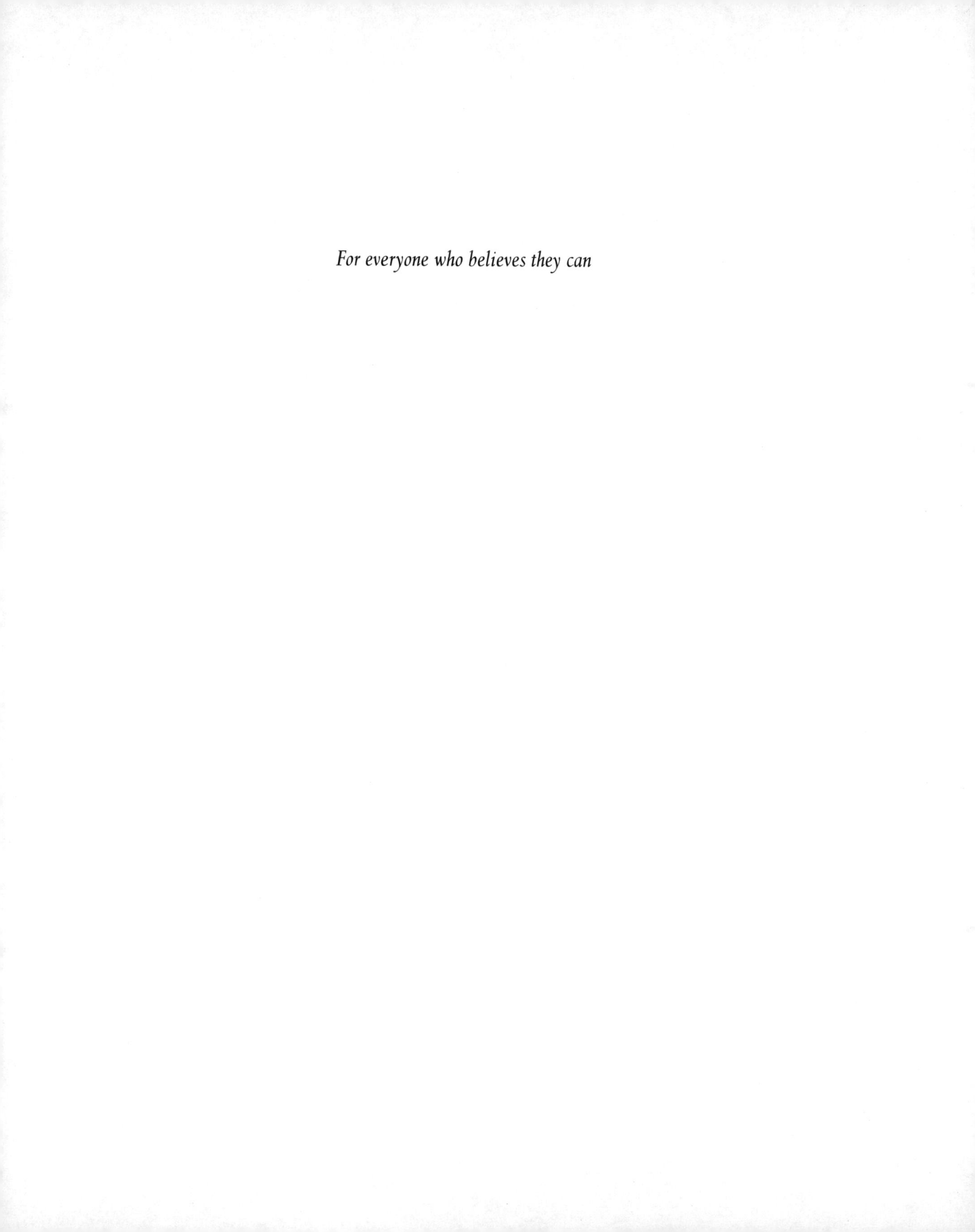

*For everyone who believes they can*

# Contents

# Introduction

Fit bodies are everywhere you look today. On the covers of magazines, in movies, on billboards, and anywhere else advertising is possible. In the world today a lot of value is placed on fitness, and everyone at one point or another has made the decision that it's time to get in shape. The problem is that a lot of people haven't found a program they can stick with. Outsiders might see this as a lack of dedication, but that's not really the case. The issue has more to do with enjoying the workout than dedication. You just can't be dedicated to something you don't absolutely love to do. And with fitness being a lifelong process, you need something you can do, love, and keep going back to.

So what do you do? The answer is simple and is based on a form of exercise that involves absolutely no impact. It isn't running, which can be stressful on the knees and joints, and it isn't strictly weight lifting, which can be problematic from head to toe if done improperly. It's swimming. And the *Get Wet, Get Fit* program of swimming, combined with the *Get Wet, Get Fit* nutrition program, is the best way to help you reach your own specific fitness goals.

The *Get Wet, Get Fit* program gives you the methods used by elite-level swimmers, simplified to show you how to mold them into a routine you enjoy and will want to continue with for the rest of your life. Take a look at the Olympics: the swimmers' bodies are reminiscent of statues from ancient Greece, symmetrical and proportionate, fit and trim. If that's the body you've wanted, now it's time to learn how to get it.

While this book is intended mostly for the individual who wants to use swimming to become healthier, it can be equally beneficial to those who are already competitive in the sport, as we include tips from Olympians who, combined, have won twenty Olympic medals. We also cover topics you may not have previously considered a vital part of your training, such as stretching and varied dry-land training. Whoever you are, in whatever shape you're in, there's something here for you.

## WHY SWIMMING?

So why swimming? It's a logical question; why not run? Cycle? Box? Why not play tennis or basketball? All of those activities are great and can definitely help get you into shape, but swimming is the only workout you'll find that's nonweightbearing and easy on the joints. Swimming can also be far more varied than running around a track or on a treadmill—especially when you take it to the beach and out into the blue ocean—and much more entertaining than cycling at your local gym or punching a heavy bag. With tennis and team sports, you have to rely on other people not only to show up, but to put in as much effort as you to make sure you get everything out of the workout that you want. And all those who are serious about getting fit know that they're often alone, and counting on other people isn't a good idea.

So what's the best option for a program that you can do on your own to reach all of your fitness goals? Swimming. All you need is a pool—found in gyms, recreation centers, private communities, aquatic facilities—the drive, and the know-how. And that's where *Get Wet, Get Fit* comes in. It is the teaching tool you need to learn everything including how to properly swim each of the four main strokes, how to adopt a proper program suited specifically to your goals, and how to maintain the proper nutrition you will need to fuel your workouts and the program that will help you change your life for the better.

The bottom line is this: Swimming is a fantastic full-body workout that can increase your endurance, build muscle mass, and improve your body composition and cardiovascular system. And swimming can be the main component of an exercise program for anyone, young or old. It can be done indoors or out, and stay fun and fresh every single day. And, with swimming, you have none of the pain that running or lifting weights every day can bring you. Yet you still have all of the positive results. In the pages of this book you'll find the first complete program written for goal-minded individuals based around the pool. Whatever you want to accomplish physically, you can do it with the help of this book and some dedication. We start with the basics, showing you how to swim properly, and we take it a step further. We offer sample workouts and show you how to suit them perfectly to your goals. If you want to move beyond the water, included as well are the best exercises you can do in a weight room and on dry land to further enhance the building of your body. To top it off, we teach you the proper nutrition to supplement your program and put the whole puzzle together. Whatever you want to do, if you believe, you can. And we're here to help.

Before you begin your training, you will want to make sure you have all the pieces in place.

To start off on the right foot, here are some specific conditions that can be helped by swimming. Everyone knows that exercise is good for you, but what if you have a particular medical condition? Can you still swim? You most certainly can.

## CHILDREN SUFFERING FROM ASTHMA

The Department of Pediatrics, University of Maryland School of Medicine, Baltimore, found that asthmatic children who were involved in a two-month, consistent program of swim training, showed "significant improvement in all clinical variables," including "symptoms, hospitalizations, emergency room visits, and school absenteeism compared with their previous medical history or to those of age-matched controls." In addition, these benefits were visible even up to a full year after the program was discontinued.

## THE ELDERLY

A Belgian study from 2003 found that low-active elderly people (fifty-five and older) not only increased their technique and speed after just five weeks of swim training but also increased flexibility in their hips, ankles, and head. The study also found increased strength in the legs, arms, and back.

A separate Japanese study from 2001 found that swimming regularly provides "increases in cardiovascular fitness (maximal oxygen consumption and endurance), muscle strength and overall functional capacity . . . allowing elderly individuals to maintain their independence, increase levels of spontaneous physical activity and freely participate in activities associated with daily living."

## HYPERTENSION PATIENTS

Researchers at the University of Tennessee–Knoxville conducted a study to find how swimming relates to hypertension patients. While it is known that swimming is a great way to prevent high blood pressure, before this 1997 study there was little to show how it helped, if it did so at all, people who already had blood pressure issues.

The team at UT found that the resting heart rates of the study patients dropped significantly after just ten weeks of aquatic training. Aside from the benefits found, which presumably can be applied to anyone, the report also stated, specifically, that swimming can be a highly useful alternative for "hypertensive patients with obesity, exercise-induced asthma, or orthopedic injuries."

## SOME SCIENCE BEHIND SWIMMING

Humans are vastly inefficient in the water compared to fish. There's a host of scientific explanations for this, but the simplest explanation is that the human body was not meant to travel quickly through water. What we as a people do when we move through water is unnatural, which makes it both a wonderful exercise and a great example of human ingenuity. Remember, swimming, unlike running, is still relatively new in the grand scheme of life.

Water is hundreds of times denser than air. It's a whole different medium that requires the body to minimize drag forces while maximizing propulsion and efficiency. It requires full-body exercise and a new management system by the body to handle a lack of oxygen as compared to exercise on solid ground.

The Counsilman Center for the Science of Swimming conducted research that found physiological markers of aging more favorable in those who swam than in those who did not. In addition, the swimmers' markers in both blood lipids (cholesterol) and blood pressure were more favorable than those of sedentary individuals. For young and old, swimming has been shown to increase muscle mass (lean tissue) while minimizing body fat (adipose tissue). Furthermore, swimming has been proven to increase flexibility and, as a result, create a more favorable physical condition for blood circulation, which then leads to increased energy and even a higher level of brain function. As you can see, on a physiological level, swimming provides a host of benefits. And all of that is aside from the fact that it's just plain fun to do.

Swimming, like any other exercise, burns calories by using stores in the body for fuel. The Counsilman Center found that when a person is swimming at a speed of less than 1 meter per second, calorie expenditure is directly related to velocity. That is to say, someone swimming at 0.5 meter per second is burning more calories than someone swimming along at 0.4 meter per second. Additionally, due to the average of higher body weight, men generally burn more calories while swimming than women, a fact that is shared across the board of physical activity.

As it is conducted in a body of water, swimming activity is considered impact-free and thus suitable for people of all types, ages, and conditions. Big or small, world-class athlete or stay-at-home parent, swimming provides a means of physical fitness for everyone.

## PREPARATION

Getting into the best shape of your life isn't exactly like playing the stock market, but there are some principles common to them both. And since understanding is important and it's easier to do with a comparison, we'll use the stock exchange.

When you're investing in the stock market, you make trades and hope for the best. You do your research; maybe you talk to some people and get what you feel is an inside scoop. Maybe you're guessing that an analyst is about to make an upgrade on a stock, and you buy hoping. Maybe you catch wind of a rumor that a company is about to upgrade its earnings estimate, and you buy, saying a prayer all the while that it will come to pass. Or perhaps those increasingly long lines at Costco give you the idea it's going to have a heck of a quarter, and you buy. Again, hoping.

Fitness isn't about hoping as the stock market is. Getting in shape isn't subject to the economy or an analyst who can publicly downgrade you, and your homework doesn't involve listening to boring conference calls. You have to be prepared for anything you do, whether it's buying a stock, losing fat, gaining muscle, or even making your breakfast. If you simplify anything enough, if it's something that has an end result, there has to be some sort of preparation. An easy example: Getting dressed? You have to get out of bed. You get the idea.

Preparing to start a fitness program has several steps:

1. Understand what your goals are.

   When you're exercising, you need to know why you're doing it. You need to know what you're doing and what it benefits, how it works, and the end result you're going for.

2. Think long-term.

   Fitness isn't like a game that can be won or lost. It's an evolving effort that you're either constantly "winning" or constantly "losing." You make short-term changes with a long-term goal in mind. The changes are short-term because improving your life doesn't stop and there's a consistent evolution in various parts of your program. It's a constant effort, something that can happen as long as you're willing to work for it.

## Olympian Tip Finding Balance with Swimming

***Val Kalmikovs—***
***two-time Olympian (Latvia) and Masters World Champion***
***Joy Kalmikovs—Australia National Team***

Balance yourself. The amount of effort you place in swimming should be the same that is applied to the rest of your life. Work hard in your swimming and fitness goals, but don't forget to play. Everyone needs to let their hair down every now and again. You'll gain better results by balancing your life and enjoying every aspect of it.

3. Have the right tools.

   This book is a great start. But there are other resources necessary. Obviously, this book talks a lot about getting in shape using a pool. So you'll need a gym that has a pool, a pool of your own, or a community/school pool you can use.

   Because fitness consists of both exercise and nutrition, you'll need the right foods and the tools to prepare them if you don't have them already.

   You don't want to get to the pool or gym mentally and physically ready and not have the right equipment. Have your water bottles, swimsuit, cap, goggles, and whatever else you'll need in hand and ready to go. One rule that remains true with physical fitness is that it's better to be overprepared than underprepared. While they are optional, if you want to really expand your training you will want to have things like a kickboard, pull buoy, and paddles on hand. We'll discuss these pieces of equipment and more later on.

4. Ignore criticism.

   Too often a well-meaning friend or family member makes a comment, a joke, or some sort of remark that isn't intended to be malicious but has a sort of negative connotation to it. What they don't realize is that people are often daunted by the work involved when it comes to getting in shape, and they take this sort of criticism very personally. Sometimes personally enough that the people on the receiving end give up on their goals.

   Almost everyone is self-conscious to a degree, but some people don't always realize what they're saying to someone they care about. Because we can't control everything that those around us say, learning to listen selectively is very beneficial. Try to limit conversations with people you know aren't always positive. If you have a negative aunt or uncle, or anyone who is just known for constant pessimism, you don't have to ignore them, but it's not a bad idea to stay on safer topics.

Remember, fitness is your personal goal and you not only can but will achieve it, if you give it the necessary effort, give it value in your life, and enjoy it.

1

# Key Concepts

Before we begin teaching the basics of each stroke, along with some tips to keep moving you forward, there are a few things that should be remembered throughout the process. First, you're probably going to be reading some things you haven't heard before even if you've been around swimming for any length of time. Many people learn a normalized way to swim in swim lessons or on high school teams. A lot of coaches at the younger levels are very good at teaching the basics but aren't able to delve too far into the finer mechanics of swimming. At the high school level, swim teams are often difficult sports to field a coach for, and many times a well-meaning teacher takes the spot just so the kids can have a place to compete. These people are giving it a heroic effort but understandably can't offer the type of instruction necessary to really teach someone how to move quickly and efficiently through the water.

Enjoy the water, play around a bit, and get used to it. It seems childish to some people at first, but it develops comfort in the water, and the water should be a comfortable place to have fun. The best thing to do when learning how to swim is to practice in some very shallow water. Don't go even shoulder high if possible. A beginning swimmer who knows he/she can stand up and be only waist deep in water will be much more relaxed than one who stands up tall and is covered to the chin.

Additionally, if you haven't swum before, remember that swimming may be a frustrating sport to pick up on. There's a lot to it, which is one of the great things about it. Because it takes so much coordination and a good amount of skill, it translates into a fantastic workout. You'll also be learning a potentially lifesaving ability that will make you more comfortable when you're at the beach, poolside at a hotel, or maybe even in your own backyard. The key is not to get discouraged and never give up. All great things take work, and learning to become a better swimmer and getting fit in the process are great things worth doing.

If you do get to a point of disappointment, we have a story that may help. Megan was nine years old when she started swimming (after having been kicked out of swim lessons a few years earlier), and she was far from what anyone would consider a natural. Her first length of a 25-yard pool took over three minutes (some of the fastest college male swimmers can do it in nine seconds). She was bad enough that the coaches of her team put her in a group where she was getting lapped, repeatedly, by four- and five-year-olds. If that wasn't frustrating enough, Megan disliked the water so much that she wanted to swim only backstroke because that way she could keep her face out of the water. Obviously, with some hard work and good teaching, Megan improved and has been setting and accomplishing many swimming goals ever since.

It doesn't matter where you are in terms of physical fitness level, and it certainly doesn't matter how old you are. If you're able to go through the motions, you'll be able to take advantage of all the wonderful benefits swimming can provide you throughout your life. We'll work with you step by step to get you where you want to be, and we'll start with the simplest of steps. If you're already a swimmer, feel free to advance to pages that suit your level. If you're brand new, this is the place to start.

## PERFECTING YOUR STROKE IN PHASES

No one is born a great swimmer. Some people are genetically blessed with longer limbs or exceptional flexibility, and a few have a natural "feel" for the water that entices them back into the pool at every given opportunity, but most of us improve through simple hard work and determination. When it comes to athletics, everything worthwhile takes hard work. Nothing is handed over freely, but that's why we feel such an incredible sense of accomplishment each time we improve on a particular stroke, swim an extra lap, or achieve a new personal best time.

When training to swim, you need two things: the right attitude and the right instruction. The attitude, of course, is up to you, but all of the instruction you'll need is right here. The key is to make sure that you're working at the right pace, mastering each step before moving on to the next, and tackling new challenges only when you're ready for them. For that reason, we've broken up the instructional components of this book into three phases. First, for readers who are just dipping a toe into the water (or those who took swim lessons as a kid but need to reacquaint themselves with the basics), we have the Beginner's lessons. Here we'll discuss the raw mechanics you'll need to get moving by breaking each stroke down step by step. For readers who are already comfortable in the water and know the basic components of the strokes but are ready to start moving more efficiently (as well as less-experienced swimmers who have already worked through the Beginner's lessons and are ready to refine what they've learned), we've provided the Intermediate lessons, designed specifically for them. In this Intermediate phase, experienced swimmers will learn how to get the best workout possible from swimming. And finally, for those readers who are interested in swimming at a more competitive or advanced level, we've included the Advanced lessons.

We'll discuss the strokes one by one, including the most common strokes, freestyle and backstroke, as well as what are called the short-axis strokes, the breaststroke and butterfly. If you're comfortable in the water and more inclined to work on a particular stroke or certain mechanics, skip around. Whatever you do, be positive and enjoy!

## THE STREAMLINE

You're going to learn a lot in the following sections. You'll learn the basics and the finer points of each stroke, and it's a lot to take in. But one thing stays constant throughout any type of swimming, and that's the "streamline." We'll talk more about it in some of these sections, but if you're going through in order, remember the following:

The streamline position is the most drag-efficient position you can be in while moving through the water. You make your body as long as possible in a straight line, extending your arms straight upward, biceps over your ears, hands overlapping. Keep your legs together, straight, and toes pointed. Practice this standing up. The sooner you get to know this position, the better. You just can't perfect it enough!

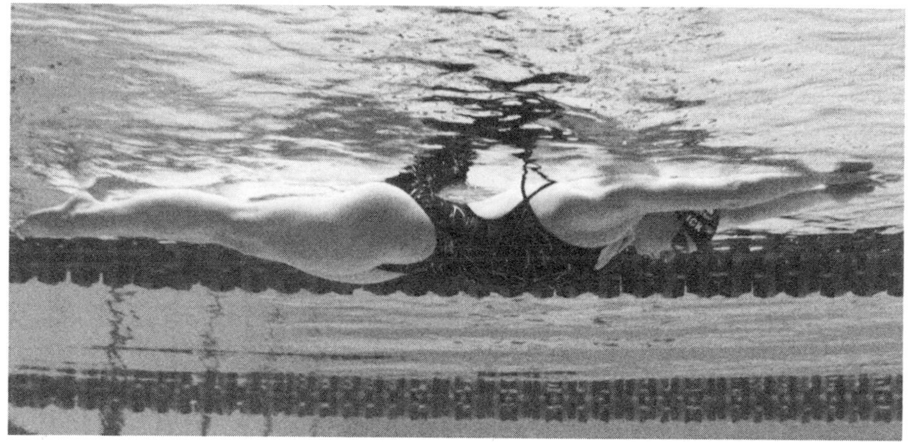

The streamline is the most drag-efficient position you can be in when swimming. You will find yourself in this position off of each start and turn, so it is very important to master it.

2

# Breaststroke

Breaststroke is a powerful strength-training and fat-burning workout packed into one stroke. Utilizing more muscle strength than the crawl or backstroke, and producing more even tone than butterfly (which focuses more on developing the muscles of the upper body), breaststroke is the "total gym" workout of the pool.

The wonderful thing about breaststroke is that it's easily adapted for all different levels of fitness—just as suitable for the serious fitness enthusiast as for the elderly or for those who just want to relax and get a bit of exercise in the pool. The body positioning of the stroke makes it fairly easy to float, very easy to move the arms and legs, to rotate the hips, and to press back and forth. No other stroke offers as many options for muscle work as breaststroke, and there's no impact, so it's easy even on a recovering body.

Breaststroke is a very easy stroke to swim and a difficult stroke to perfect, but because it uses so many different muscle groups you'll get a terrific total-body workout while you learn. As with any stroke, you'll want to start by becoming well versed in the basic elements and then, after you're comfortable, work on building speed and power.

## BEGINNER'S BREASTSTROKE

Breaststroke is propelled by the arms, using a pulling motion toward the body, and a froglike kick of the legs. To begin, you float facedown in the water, in the streamline position, with your arms extended straight in front of you and your legs extended straight behind you. From this starting point, breaststroke can be broken down into six simple steps:

1. Keeping your elbows on top of the water—just shy of breaking the surface—bend from the elbow down (the half from the elbow to your fingertips) as if you were pointing your fingers straight down toward the bottom of the pool. Move your elbows outward a bit (similar to making a Y shape with your body). Begin pulling back toward your body.

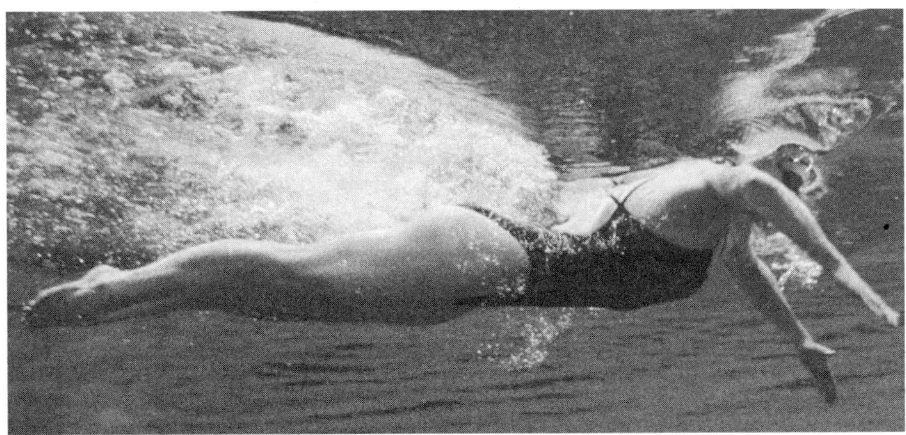

The elbows stay up in breaststroke, which allows a swimmer to use the entire forearm to pull water, rather than simply the backs of the arms, which is what happens if the elbows drop.

2. While beginning step 1 and keeping your legs close together (knees about eight to ten inches apart), bend at the knees, bringing your heels toward your back.

3. As your arms pull back to the point where your elbows become in line with your nose—making sure your elbows stay near the surface of the water—bend at the elbows and bring your palms together under your chest, with your palms overlapping.

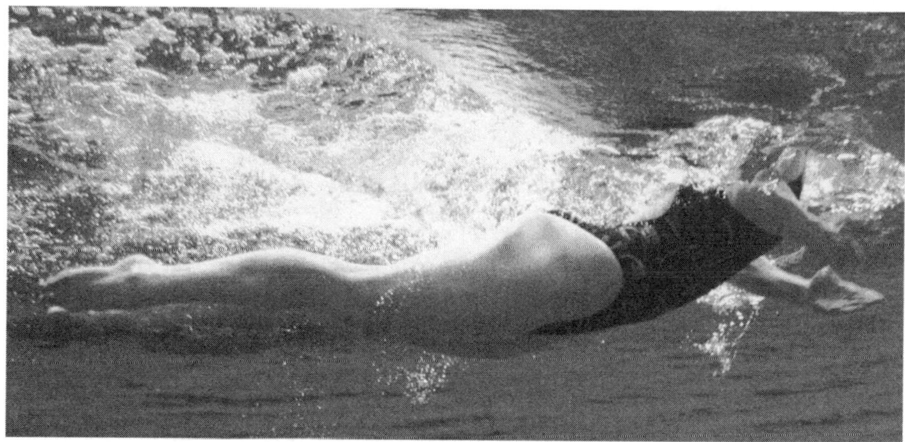

Finishing the pull in breaststroke is about quickness. Move the hands quickly under the chest and forward, making sure there's no pause as the hands come together.

4. Simultaneously kick apart and out with your legs (like the kick of a frog) and thrust your hands forward, fully extending your arms.

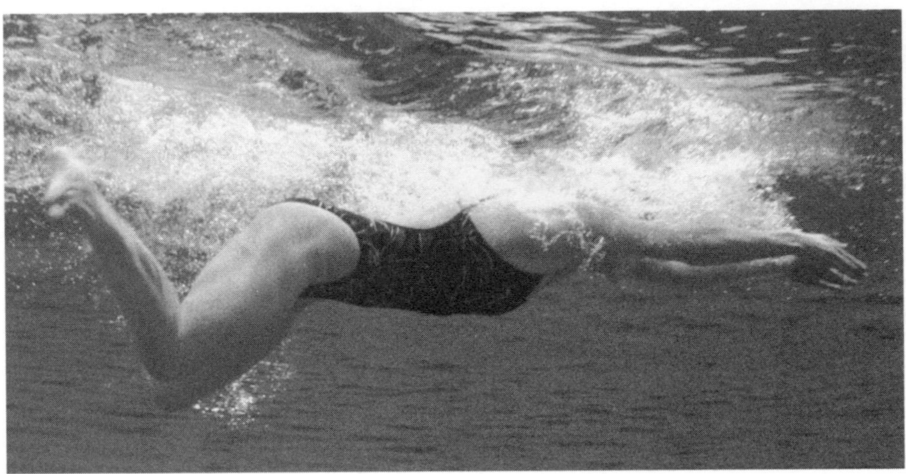

As the hands fully extend forward, the legs kick back powerfully. Toes should be pointed to the sides of the pool to ensure that the whole bottom of the foot is used to push water.

5. Finish the kick so that the legs come back together and fully extend the whole body, returning to your starting position.

6. Allow the body to glide through the water, and once you begin to slow down, repeat from step 1. If this is your first time trying this stroke, congratulations, you've just swum breaststroke!

In addition to learning the mechanics of the stroke, there are a few things you should keep in mind:

- Enjoy the glide! One of the greatest aspects of swimming is that it makes you feel weightless and free. The glide is the movement you get to enjoy after pulling and kicking, so use it to recover before your next pull and kick.
- As you kick and thrust your arms forward to extension, do so

quickly. If you pause while your arms are underneath your body, your hips will begin to sink and it will become more difficult to kick. Keep everything fluid and without pausing during each stroke.

- If you drop your elbows while stroking, you'll be pulling with only the back of your upper arms (your triceps) and you'll be pulling much less water, as well as using far fewer muscles. Be sure to keep your elbows near the surface of the water so you're able to pull the water with your palms and forearms.

Above all, have fun. As with any fitness program, you'll stick with it only if you're enjoying yourself, so don't push yourself too hard. Even if you move slowly at first, you'll be getting in shape, so go at your own pace and enjoy the process.

## Common Mistakes to Avoid

Many people think so much about what they need to do right, they sometimes overlook other things. We're including a few things that you may not specifically consider but are definitely worth thinking about next time you're in the pool.

Breaststroke is as difficult as it is simple. That may sound confusing, but it's true. When something is as simple as breaststroke, there are a lot of ways to just get through it rather than doing it well. By saying that, we mean it's very easy to lift your head, swirl your arms, kick your legs, and throw your head back underwater and repeat. But it is hard to execute an efficient, well-formed stroke. As you're working to improve the many facets of breaststroke, there are some common mistakes you will want to make sure you're not getting into the habit of making.

First, make sure you're not just lifting your chin to breathe. A lot of new breaststrokers pull their chin back so far it looks as if they're trying to examine the ceiling.

Next, be sure you're pushing back with your kick and not simply out. Concentrate on actually kicking water behind you for propulsion.

Finally, don't bend your wrists. In fact, think of your arm as solid and flat from the elbow down.

## INTERMEDIATE BREASTSTROKE

By this point you're able to complete several laps fluidly and you're ready to start picking up some speed. So without further ado, let's improve your stroke!

You can use the following tips in any order you prefer, so feel free to choose the aspects of the stroke you're most interested in working on. If you feel like refining one aspect of your stroke for several workouts in a row until you see an improvement, that's just fine, and once that element improves you'll be in a better position to improve the next part. No one has a perfect stroke, and everyone modifies the stroke slightly to make it work for him or her, so feel free to experiment a bit.

### Head Position

When swimming breaststroke, the most common thing to do is to look forward toward the other side of the pool. It's human nature to want to look where you're going. In breaststroke, though, lifting the chin so that your eyes can see ahead of you will alter the position of your spine. When you're swimming this stroke, keep your head in the same position as if you were walking upright. To get the exact feel, sit against a wall with your back and head flat against it. Look straight ahead. This is the position you want to maintain at all times when swimming breaststroke. Notice in the following picture how Megan's head is in line with her back.

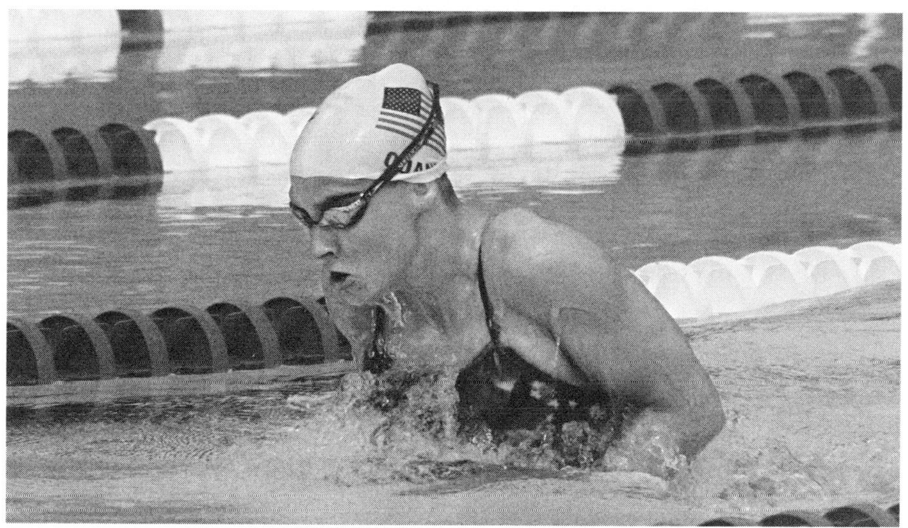

Head position can affect any stroke but can make it especially hard to swim proper breaststroke. Keep the head in line with the spine just as if you were walking upright.

## Hand Movement

As you're kicking and pushing your hands forward to get into your glide position, keep your hands at the surface of the water. If they are too low, you'll create drag, slowing yourself down. If they are too high—out of the water—your uneven weight distribution will cause your body to sink and, even worse, cause you to waste energy, which will further slow you later.

### Kick

As you've discovered by now, the power of this stroke really comes from the kick. In order to get the most out of each kick, turn the bottoms of your feet inward and clap them together (like you would clap the palms of your hands) just as you're reaching full extension. There are stories that some male Olympic breaststrokers have finished their kicks so powerfully that they bruised the bottoms of their feet!

Improvement often comes in small steps, and with each small modification you perfect, you'll find it easier to incorporate the other refinements. For example, when your head is in the proper position, your body will be better aligned to push your hands forward *and* press your kick back. Likewise, when you are pushing your hands forward at the correct level, your hips are more likely to be posi-

#### Olympian Tip — Breaking Down the Kick

***Ed Moses—***
***gold and silver medalist, 2000 Sydney Olympics***

The biggest jump in my career in breaststroke was when I really broke down my kick and analyzed it. I made huge stroke and time improvements when I moved to a more dynamic, compact kick. Instead of allowing my knees to drift outward and underneath my body, I kept my knees closer together and pulled my heels to my butt instead of bringing my knees toward my chest. This allowed me to stay in a position of less drag and still maintain a powerful and supportive kick. A great drill for this is kicking breaststroke on your back with a buoy between your legs and not letting your knees break the surface of the water.

tioned just as you need them so you can kick powerfully. Little improvements add up quickly. So be proud of each and every improvement! Even if you've been swimming this stroke since your summer camp days, it's never too late to become more efficient.

## ADVANCED BREASTSTROKE

In competitive swimming, height is usually a very important factor in assisting speed. Such swimming greats as Olympians Michael Phelps (6'4"), Ian Crocker (6'4"), and Gary Hall Jr. (6'6") stand tall among the competition on the men's side, and even the majority of great female swimmers are tall compared to the average American woman: twenty-six-time national champion and multiple Olympian Jenny Thompson stands 5'10", and Olympian Courtney Shealy stands 6'3". And although there are plenty of breaststroke specialists (such as Olympian Kristy Kowal and German national team member and World University Games medalist Janne Schaefer) who stand taller than six feet, breaststroke is one of the few strokes that gives those who are less genetically blessed in height a chance to shine.

As a sixteen-year-old, Megan competed in the finals of the 100-meter breaststroke at the Olympic Games in Sydney, Australia. She was the fastest American woman in the world that year up to that point, and on that night she was the fastest once again, winning the gold medal for America. Just days later, she climbed back onto the blocks as a member of the American 4 x 100-meter medley relay team that smashed the world record, becoming the first women's medley relay team ever to go under four minutes. That day Megan swam the fastest 100-meter breaststroke time a woman had ever swum, even though at 5'7", Megan was one of the shortest swimmers at the Olympics.

How exactly has Megan overcome her relatively small stature to win so many awards for breaststroke? She focuses on developing two key facets: efficient power and explosiveness. In order to achieve power and explosiveness in your own breaststroke, there are three things that you'll want to keep in mind. These three aspects of swimming breaststroke are the same whether you're going for Olympic gold, for a more aesthetic physique, or for a fitter cardiovascular system. They are:

1. Start and finish each stroke in the streamline position.
2. When pulling, use the path of *most* (beneficial) resistance.
3. Always use a "three-step" kick.

It's difficult to incorporate all three of these modifications into your stroke at the same time, so in the following paragraphs we'll break each one of them down separately, explaining how it will help your swimming, no matter what your goal is.

### 1. Start and finish each stroke in the streamline position.

Except for your last stroke each length, each movement in breaststroke is followed immediately by the next. The goal is to draw the most possible force from the previous stroke to propel you forward with the next, moving your energy forward. To do this, you want to create as little drag as possible against the water, and the key is to extend and lock your arms and legs, with one hand over the other, your biceps pressed over the ears. Swimmers refer to this position as the "streamline," and it's vital between strokes because it creates the least amount of drag possible as the body moves through water. If the arms are not straight and the elbows, shoulders, and back flare out, there is more body surface working against the water to slow you down and create drag. The same approach applies to your leg position. If your knees are bent and out of alignment with the rest of your body, the water is able to press against you and hold you back. Many swimmers also point their toes when assuming the streamline in the water.

For the fitness swimmer not concerned with speed, the streamline is still vital to overall development of the muscles. Why? Because it is the optimal starting point to recruit every muscle as you go through the stroke. If you start and finish each stroke with bent limbs, your muscles won't be used to their fullest extent. For example, if the pull portion of the stroke is started and finished with the hands outside the shoulder line (imagine two straight lines starting on top of your shoulders and continuing directly upward), the deltoids and forearms are both being partially neglected. One of the major benefits of swimming for fitness is that it makes it very easy to work the whole body if done properly, so you don't want to limit your range of motion.

### 2. When pulling, use the path of *most* (beneficial) resistance.

Most swimmers are used to hearing that their primary concern, from the moment they enter the water, is to avoid creating resistance. And it's true that you want to minimize the drag on your body going through the water, but there are times you can use resistance, which is different from drag, to your advantage. To understand the difference, imagine that you're paddling a boat. It's difficult to pull the oar through the water because there's resistance against it. But you're using this resistance to move you forward. Drag, instead, is like attaching an anchor to your boat. With drag, there's more surface area, which stops you from gliding through the water easily and thus slows you down.

When you pull with breaststroke, bending at the elbows and drawing your arms back in toward your body, you want to feel resistance on the inside portion of your hands and forearms just as if they were the oars that are paddling your boat. Most often, coaches are so set on preaching "No Resistance" that they miss making a vital distinction: When pulling, you're not creating drag, you're using resistance, just as you would when moving a boat from one end of a lake to another.

The idea when swimming breaststroke is to pull on the water

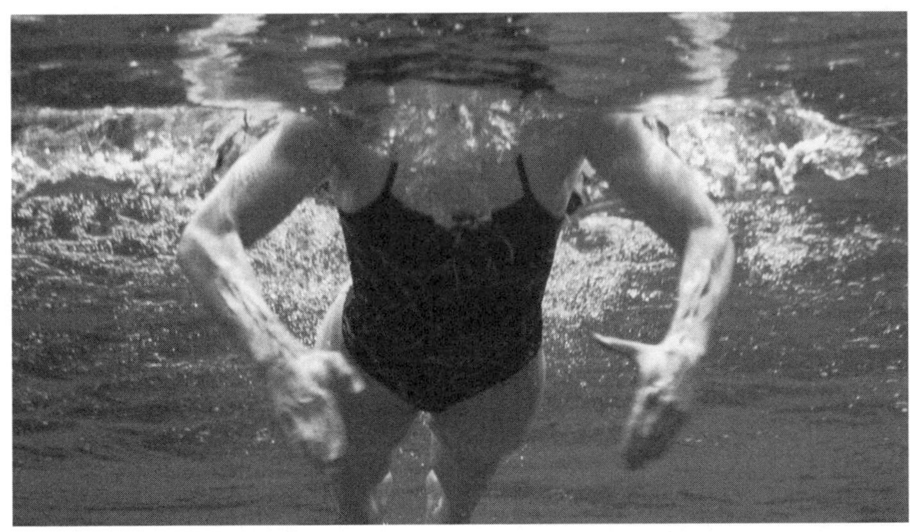

Be sure not to bend at the wrists when pulling. Keep your arms in one line from the elbow all the way down to the end of your fingertips.

with your upper body and kick the water away so that you propel yourself forward. If you take a stroke and feel as if you're not pulling on anything, then you're taking the path of *least* resistance (as if you were trying to paddle that boat with the thin portion of the oar). This feels easier, but it doesn't work the muscles and doesn't move you very quickly. When you pull with your arms, you want to keep your elbows up and your forearm, wrist, and hand in one straight line from your elbow down. As you pull back, you'll feel the pressure of your movement against the water: paddling with the big side of the oar. This is what you want—to pull as much water as possible and take the path of *most* resistance *inward.* Drag is the outward component—the anchor—you should try to avoid.

**3. Always use a three-step kick.**

The breaststroke kick is usually the first kick that children learn when going through swim lessons. It's more commonly known to them as the frog kick, and it was one of the main methods of propulsion used when modern swimming competitions began in the 1800s. There is a trick to doing the frog kick in the most effective way. What many children don't learn is that there are actually three parts to each kick. The difference between the kicks of good swimmers and the best swimmers is usually very evident in underwater video footage. Megan's kicks, for example, always follow the same pattern:

1. She brings her heels up to her backside, ensuring she keeps her knees close.

2. She turns her feet out so that her toes are pointed toward the sides of the pool.

3. She presses the bottoms of her feet directly behind her to "kick" the water and finishes in a circular motion to bring the feet together.

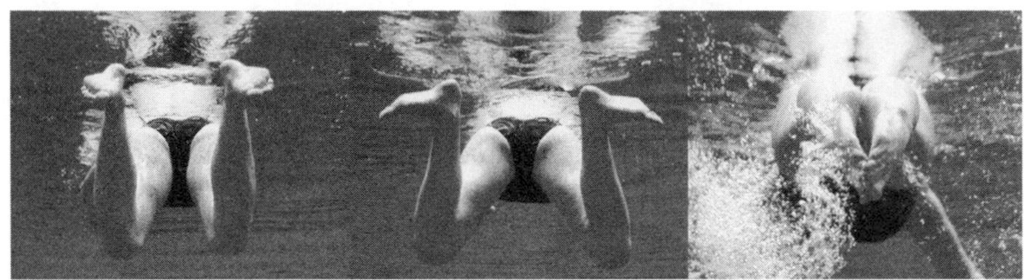

The progression of the kick. Pull the heels back, turn the toes out, and push the water back as you kick, ending with your feet together. If your feet don't touch, you're losing precious power.

As we mentioned earlier when we talked about finishing each stroke in the same position, you need to streamline your kick. To get the most use out of the legs and to involve as much muscle as possible, you need to ensure you're following the steps laid out above. As the pull begins, you bring your heels up behind you. In the interest of preventing drag and aligning properly, you want to keep your knees fairly close together—about eight to ten inches apart on average (more for extremely tall people)—and widen only slightly, roughly another couple of inches, as the feet push against the water and out. As the kick progresses, the legs move in a half-circular motion as they round out and the feet touch at the end. Then the streamline is resumed, and the process begins again.

3

# Freestyle

Also known as the "crawl stroke," this is the most commonly swum stroke in lap pools all around the world. Whereas the term "freestyle" in a race description really just means you can swim any stroke—a free choosing of a style of stroke—it has long been used to describe the front crawl.

The freestyle is the fastest stroke in the water and is fairly simplistic in nature. It involves simple, instinctive motions that people feel natural doing when in the water: kicking with legs extended and pulling the length of the body. The stroke works numerous muscles, but particularly the triceps, core, and legs.

As you may have seen from watching Olympic swimmers, or even some swimmers at your local pool, the ones who look the most relaxed are usually the fastest and most technically sound. Swimming is a beautiful exercise, and it's beautiful in the sense that it's somewhat like art. Gliding through the water while causing little disturbance (swimming without splashing wildly and without slapping the water) is a part of great swimming. It's a sight to see, and people are amazed by it. If you follow these steps, people will be impressed by your skills—and by your physique because of the great workout you'll be getting each time you practice.

Freestyle is also the easiest stroke to vary your intensity with. You can go right into sprinting—giving your full effort with increased stroke rate—which will raise your heart rate; you can plug in some kicking drills and pulling drills; you can gain comfort by the ease you have with floating since your body is elongated. There are so many benefits to learning this set of skills.

After dedicated practice and workouts, an additional benefit—aside from that appealing "summer body" all year long—is that you'll know a potentially lifesaving skill. What you learn here isn't just for the pool, it's for the ocean or the lake—any body of water.

## BEGINNER'S FREESTYLE

Most people, if thrown in a pool when they're not sure how to swim, will thrash violently at the water one arm at a time, head up, leaning slightly forward. Naturally, problems ensue with this because the body isn't at an angle that allows it to pass smoothly through water. The drag created by a vertical body can hardly be overcome by two arms. As such, proper freestyle is swum in an efficiently flat position.

The proper body position when swimming freestyle is much like that of the body when standing up straight, with a few minor changes. One of the more important things to remember is that your head should remain, except when breathing, in the same position when you're in the water as it is when you're standing out of it.

When starting the freestyle stroke, you should be in the "streamline" position. The streamline is when you're extending your arms straight over your head, pressing your biceps over your ears, and placing one hand on top of the other. In addition to that, just point your toes as straight as possible, and you've got it. When done properly, the streamline is the most drag-efficient position the body can be in while moving through the water. Races start in this position, and turns off of every wall use it as well. It's an important position to master, and as you continue to get better at it—keeping your arms in tighter, keeping your back flat—you'll quickly realize how much smoother you are in the water.

Follow these steps for your pulling phase:

1. From the streamline position, bring one arm just outside the shoulder line and bend at the elbow so that your fingers are pointing to the bottom of the pool.

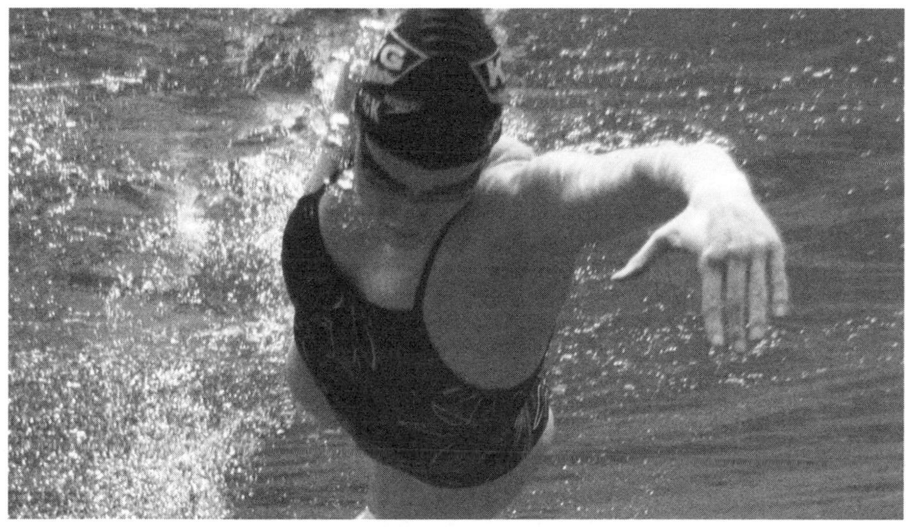

The elbow shouldn't drop when the freestyle pull is started. Keeping the arm up, just bend from the elbow down toward your fingers.

Pull back with the same arm, and as it passes the hips, fully extend the arm (you should feel your triceps flex at extension).

2. Bend the same arm at the elbow and bring it forward, back toward your initial streamline position. Bring your elbow high out of the water so that your fingers clear the surface. This is called, simply, a high-elbow recovery.

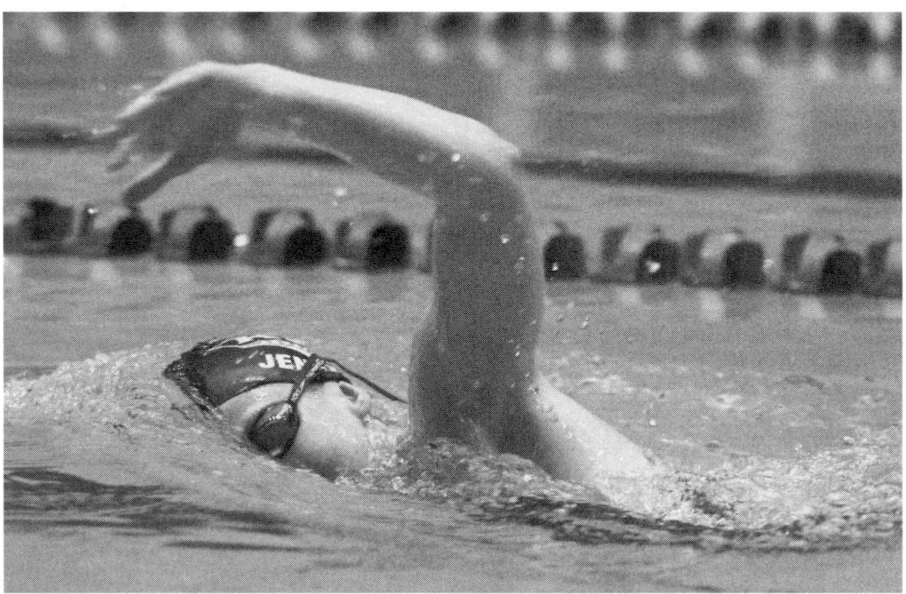

There are a lot of ways to complete a freestyle stroke, the most common being a high-elbow recovery.

3. At the same time, repeat step 1 with your other arm, and continue to do so in an alternating pattern. If you just swam freestyle for the first time, great job!

When swimming, you should also have a strong kick behind you. Point your toes and have your knees bent just slightly. Kick with the length of your leg, beginning at the hips, and not just from the knee down.

Breathing while swimming the freestyle is done during the recovery phase—the portion when you are bringing your arm in front of you again—and is a simple, single motion to one side of the body. As the arm is recovering, turn your head to the same side, just enough to bring your mouth clear of the water, take in a breath, and return the head to its regular facedown position.

Taking a breath for a new swimmer can be a bit difficult at first. Resist the urge to bring your head up completely to get air. Doing so throws off the body alignment and makes it much more difficult to propel through the water. Just follow the steps slowly and relax. One of the secrets of good swimming is knowing when to relax the body and knowing when to tense it up. For the enthusiast and fitness swimmer, knowing when to relax is much, much more important at this point. Tensing of the muscles is used for power techniques, and right now we're simply working on getting through the water smoothly.

## Common Mistakes to Avoid

One easy mistake that most people make is having their head position too high. By saying "high" we're referring to having your head pulled back and keeping much of your forehead out of the water as you swim. Remember, this will push your hips down and make it harder to rotate properly.

It's also very important to keep an eye on your pull. Are you overreaching? Ask yourself this question often and check up on it. This is one of the simplest ways to immediately improve your swimming.

While you're thinking about where your pull is starting, also think about where it's finishing. Remember the analogy of where your body is strongest, and apply that. If you're pulling underneath your body, down your center line, you're getting far less propulsion than if you were to pull just outside of the body, in the same line as your hand entered.

Finally, always be kicking! By far the most chronic problem among freestyle swimmers of all ages is an inconsistent kick. If you step on the gas in your car only every few seconds, you're going to have a pretty rough, and slow, ride. Likewise, if you're kicking only every few strokes, it's going to be a much harder session in the pool. A continuous kick allows the body to ride higher, smoother, and faster.

## INTERMEDIATE FREESTYLE

As you've seen, the front crawl is a stroke that, on the basic level, has only a few steps and, once you get the hang of it, is quite simple. As always, there are some things that can be done to further refine and improve your stroke. If you're able to move about the pool comfortably doing this freestyle stroke, then you're ready to move on. If you want to really clean up your stroke and cut smoothly through the water, try following some of these tips.

## Head Position

Keep your head in line with the rest of your body. You can look up at your hand from underwater to check the entry of your stroke, but unless you're swimming in an open-water event or just working out in open water, that should be the only time your head is forward.

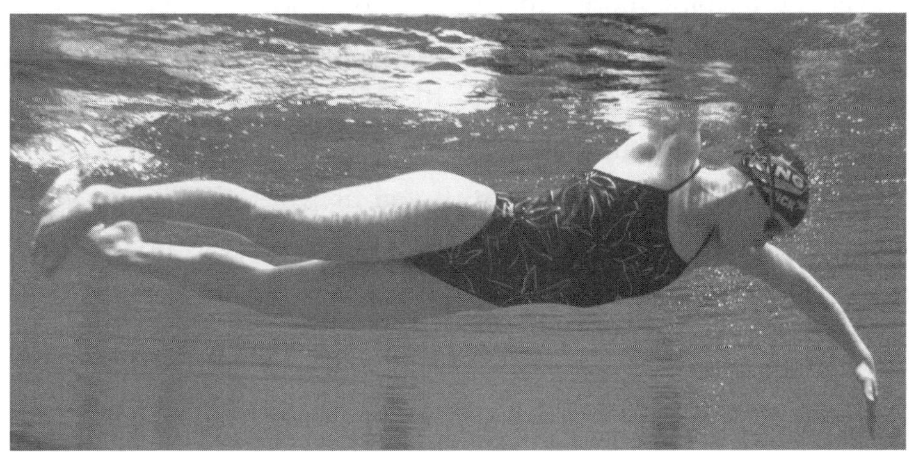

It is very important not to lift your head to look forward in freestyle. Keep your body position in line and relax your neck, focusing your eyes directly below you.

## Hand Entry

Don't splash as you enter the water with each hand. It isn't something that you notice easily when you're swimming, because most people focus simply on going through the motions, and their head is underwater. Try to enter the water with your hand straight and steady. Enter with your fingertips first and follow that entry point with the rest of your hand.

One easy way to see it is simply to look at your hand from underwater as you enter. You can also just stand up and take some practice strokes while standing still and get a feel for how the hand should be getting into the water. In swimming, smooth equals fast, and if you're causing a lot of bubbles by slapping the water, it will slow you down and take away from the efficiency of your stroke.

As you become more experienced, you'll know where the "T" (the black line on the bottom of the pool that splits off at the end of each length) is in relation to the wall, and you'll even be able to do your flip turns without looking up.

Alignment is very important. If you lift your chin, your spine can change your body position and you won't be in as straight a line as possible anymore. If your hips go down in the water, it causes more drag and makes it harder to swim. Stay looking down to keep your line. Ask any competitive swimmer, and she'll tell you she has gotten to know the bottom of the pool very well!

## Pull

Picture yourself flying, arms out in front of you in a "Superman" pose. Now picture yourself doing that in the water. If you're streamline in the water but with your arms extending straight up from your shoulders, that is the line you want to follow with your pull.

A common problem coaches of all ages see is that swimmers tend to enter with their hands in line over their heads. This changes your body position and will negatively affect your pull and is called "overreaching." Think about where you're strongest. Your back is stronger than your shoulders; if you're pulling from the line above your head, you're taking your back mostly out of the equation. If you're pulling in line with your shoulder, you'll feel much stronger because you're able to use stronger muscles.

As you pull, pay extra attention to bending your arm at the elbow, pointing your fingers directly toward the bottom of the pool while keeping your elbow high. Pull just outside of the body all the way down the length of your frame and fully extend your arm on each pull. That's called "finishing" your pull, and we'll mention it throughout the book. It's easy to shortchange yourself, your muscles, and your speed by not finishing each pull, but it's very important that you make a habit of doing it correctly.

## Kick

Your kick should be a full-lower-body effort. The movement of the leg and foot against the water is what pushes the water behind you

### Olympian Tip — Three Freestyle Tips

***Dana Vollmer—***

***gold medalist, 2004 Athens Olympics, world record holder***

- Focus on body positioning in the water. Keep a straight line and don't break it (doing so increases drag).
- Rotation is critical; don't forget to rotate while grabbing as much water as you can.
- Keep your kicks small, tight, and fast.

and causes you to move forward. Many recreational swimmers kick only from the knee down because it's easy to bend there and simply flicker the foot up and down. Your quadriceps muscles (those that make up the front, upper half of your leg) are extremely strong, though, and should definitely be a part of your kick, so long as they don't overpower it.

As you're swimming, make an effort to kick from the hips downward. Use your whole leg in the kicking motion. Your hips will, and should, move slightly left-to-right as you continue kick-

Olympian Tip **Freestyle Wisdom from an Olympic Legend**

***Gary Hall Jr.—***
***ten-time medalist, 1996 Atlanta, 2000 Sydney, 2004 Athens Olympics***

There are many fine changes in freestyle that have taken place over my swimming career. When I was taught to swim, we were told to swim with our head up, with the water surface at eyebrow level. It wasn't that long ago that everyone was taught this head position.

I remember having a conversation with Tom Jager (three-time Olympian, five gold medals) about head position. "You swim with your head up and it channels water underneath your body. Look at the front of a boat, the way a bow tapers up." It made sense to me.

Alex Popov (Olympic gold medalist, 50-meter freestyle world record holder) gets the credit for changing this. While there are others who probably started swimming with their head down before Alex, he was the one whom coaches studied and learned from and then taught their swimmers to imitate. Now most swimmers swim with their head down, and faster.

ing. This movement will build a strong cadence for your kick, and this simple change will be one of the easiest ways to improve your swimming.

## ADVANCED FREESTYLE

### Arm Movement

A lot of swimmers use what is called a "catch-up" stroke, which is where one arm stays streamline nearly the entire time the other arm is going through the pull and moves only once the other arm has returned back to streamline. Athletes like Olympian Ian Thorpe can swim phenomenally fast with a longer stroke, whereas most swimmers keep their arms at specific distances from each other. In time, you will find what is best for you, but here we talk basics.

When moving your arms in the pulling motions, you should think of them as needing to be opposites. For example, when your right arm is completely extended at the finishing point of its pull, your left arm should be completely extended in front of you. As the right arm moves, you then begin moving the left. Optimally, when using a strong kick and keeping your body in a proper alignment, your right arm will be at its highest recovery point above your shoulder as your left arm is directly below.

### Finish the Stroke Through to the Hips

Most strokes end when the pulling gets tough; it's quite easy to pull down to the stomach, lift the elbow out of the water, and start over. It's easy because you're able to use quite a bit of momentum and body weight. If you do this, though, you leave a lot of force behind.

When pulling, make each pull count for all it's worth. Pull the full length of your body, which means extending your arms—and using your triceps to their fullest extent—past the hips on each stroke cycle.

## Pro Tip Important Components of Sprinting

***Nick Brunelli—***
***gold medalist, 2003 Pan American Games; gold and bronze medalist, 2004 Short Course World Championships***

Many swimmers think the faster you move your arms through the water, the faster you will go. That's not necessarily true when sprinting. The first thing that needs to be done to become faster in sprint events is to forget about creating power with every stroke. The idea of sprinting is to maximize your efficiency by reducing drag just as in any other event. However, adding a higher stroke rate and a hard kick makes it very difficult to hold that efficient stroke you may have when swimming slowly. Here are a few ideas to help hold your stroke while adding tempo.

In order to swim as efficiently as possible, you first need to put your body in perfect alignment. To do this, imagine yourself swimming in the pool with a pole extending out from the farthest wall (where the surface of the water and the wall meet), extending all the way down the length of the pool and through the center of your forehead. Then imagine that pole extending through your center core all the way down to your feet and continuing out to the other end of the pool, behind you. This imaginary pole represents a perfectly flat solid line that doesn't ever move. This line now becomes the exact line you will need to swim on in order to be in perfect alignment. As you swim, you will, of course, need to make various movements like rotating your hips and shoulders or taking a breath. But remember that imaginary pole and do not stray away from that straight line. If you continue to swim on this line, you will automatically limit your motion left and right and up and down. You will move through the water more like a speedboat rather than a large, heavy cargo ship.

The next thing to think about while sprinting is not to rush the front part of your stroke. The most important part of a pull is the catch, which is right when your hand enters the water out front. In freestyle, when swimmers attempt to raise their stroke rate, the natural tendency is to skip this part of the stroke. When this happens, you create more of a downward entry into the water and drag air bubbles through the pull. Those air bubbles limit how much water you can hold. Successful sprinters can add tempo by increasing their stroke rate but not losing their catch, and that's why they hold so much water and move so fast.

When focusing on improving your turns, remember to be aggressive. Many people look at a turn as an obstacle and will slow down coming into a turn. I like to think of my turns as a weapon I can use to help win the race. Attack from the flags into your turn and rip your feet over quickly. Make sure your feet hit the wall no wider than hip width and strive for a great push. Think of jumping off the floor and reaching for the sky as high as possible.

4

# Backstroke

*Backstroke is the* second most commonly swum stroke, but in several ways, it is the easiest to perform. Many swimmers are comfortable with swimming long distances of backstroke because of the "easy access" to air. Whereas many people have an issue with rotating to breathe, swimming backstroke takes that obstacle away. Fortunately, while being so easy to swim and learn, backstroke is also a great workout.

## BEGINNER'S BACKSTROKE

Being comfortable with floating on your back is important to swimming backstroke. If you're at ease with that, you're set to move on to actually swimming while looking toward the ceiling or the sky.

Backstroke is simple in function. While floating on your back, begin your pull with either arm in a windmill motion, going counterclockwise, that will bring your hand over your head and behind you. While doing these steps, be sure to maintain a consistent flutter kick with your legs.

## Pull

Enter your pull in line with your shoulder.

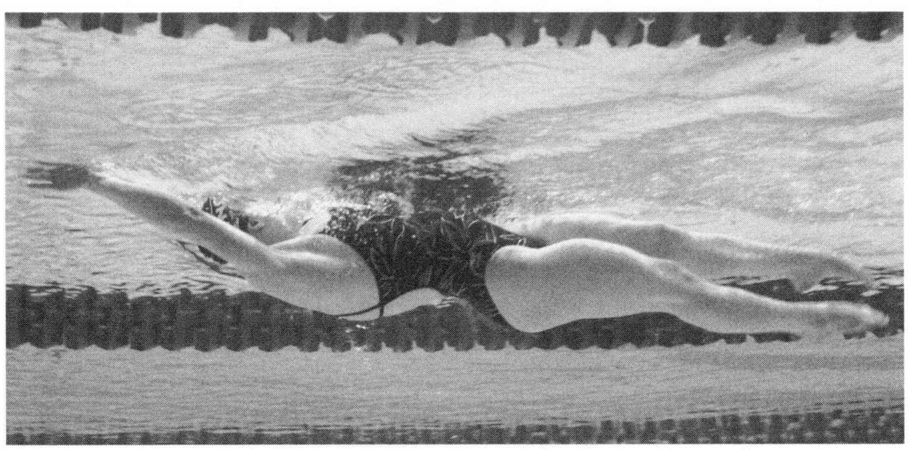

Each stroke on backstroke begins with a straight arm entering the water, ensuring that it is in line with the shoulder and not with the head or outside of the body line entirely.

Don't overreach, extending past your center line, the "imaginary" line down the exact middle of your body. Think about using your arm to pull as much water as possible; rotate so that you're able to use your whole hand and forearm to push water rather than just slicing through it.

## Kick

Think of your kick as being just like the kick you use when swimming freestyle, only upside down and smaller and faster. Use your entire leg, starting the kick at the hip, and maintain a kick throughout swimming.

### Common Mistakes to Avoid

Try not to overreach. It is very easy in backstroke to simply throw the arm back and not pay much attention to exactly where it's going. Good swimmers, however, are always very mindful of their hand entry because they know it's the beginning of a powerful pull. Make sure you're not passing your center line. Keep the hand in line with the shoulder each time it enters the water on a stroke.

Next, avoid extra-large kicking. A kick that's too big or too long can be as problematic as one that's too short or too slow. Don't bend so much at the knee that your shin is close to vertical. Your knee should be bent just slightly.

Finally, keep your kick consistent. It's easy to get caught up in just pulling your way through the backstroke, but you want to have a continuous, flowing kick. Keep the legs moving at an even rhythm, with the same number of kicks per cycle. Don't start and stop kicking at random times; make sure the movement is regular and smooth.

After trying these steps, be proud of yourself, you just swam backstroke!

---

## INTERMEDIATE BACKSTROKE

### Pull

As you're pulling your body through the water, point your fingers toward the side of the pool and drop your elbow slightly so that you can put more power into the stroke—almost like you're arm wrestling. You should feel pressure on your forearms.

Backstroke seems very simple, and it certainly is, but as with all techniques there are ways to improve and become more efficient. As you do so, you will find that you can swim faster and longer.

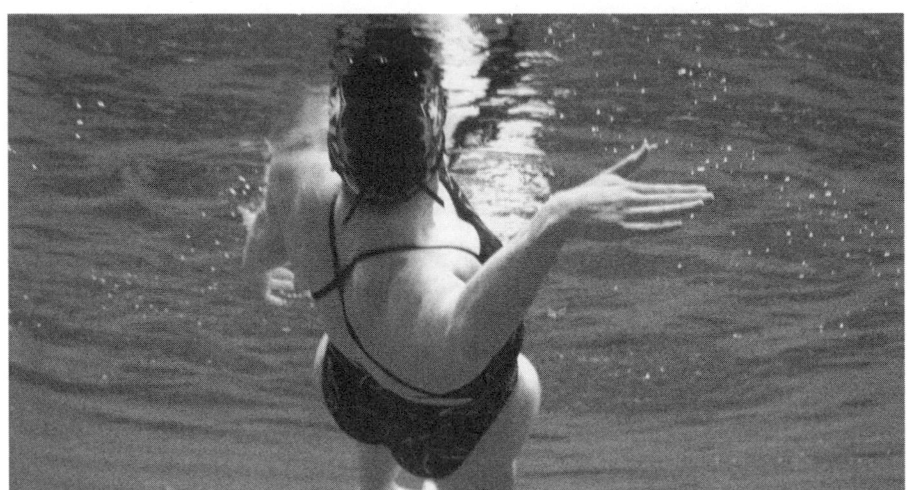

When the entry is properly placed—lining up with the shoulder—bending at the elbow and getting the proper pulling position are much easier to accomplish.

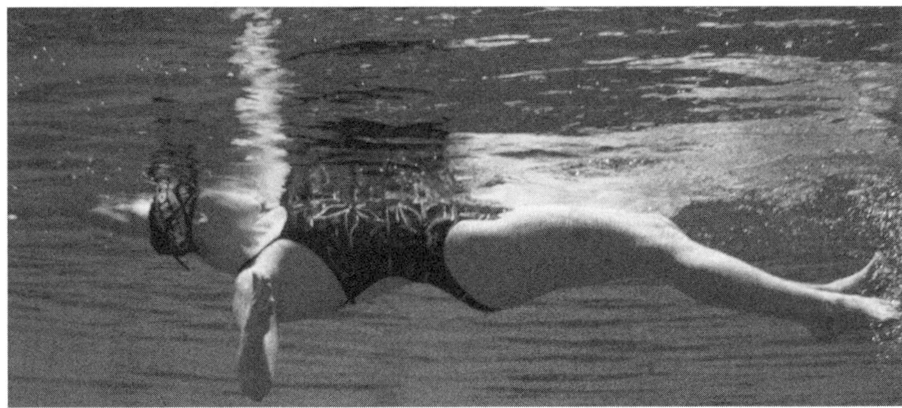

Pointing the fingers to the side of the pool with your arm in one solid line from your elbow down allows you to make use of your entire arm with each pull.

### Rotation

Good backstrokers maintain a solid rotation. Except for the head, the entire body has at least some rotation to it; when the hand is over the shoulder, the shoulder should drop and roll around rather than simply turning your hand.

## ADVANCED BACKSTROKE

Sometimes the slightest changes can make the biggest differences. Once you're comfortable swimming with fluid motion for long durations, you're set to tackle the finest points of backstroke.

Olympian Tip **Backstroke Body Position**

***Val Kalmikovs—***
***two-time Olympian (Latvia); gold medalist, Masters World Champion***
***Joy Kalmikovs—Australian National Team***

In backstroke, don't arch your back and push your chest up to keep your hips up, as this will cause your legs to sink and your hips to drop further—you'll end up swimming in the shape of a capsized boat. Instead, bend like a banana from the top of your abdominal muscles and tuck your bottom under. This will help keep your hips high and legs afloat and keep you swimming in the shape of an upright—(and hopefully fast)—boat. Keep your head still, in a neutral position.

### Kicking

Point your toes and "flick" your foot at the end of each kick. Think of your leg as an oar that you use when rowing a boat. If it is in the water and you hold it vertical, moving it up and down won't do you much good. Placing it horizontal, though, creating a large surface area to push water with, you'll build up force to propel you. Your kick should feel similar to kicking off your shoe.

### Rotation

As you're rotating your body into each stroke, finish your arm stroke down by your hips before rotating to the other side. As one arm is finishing, the other will just be entering; think of them as exact opposites.

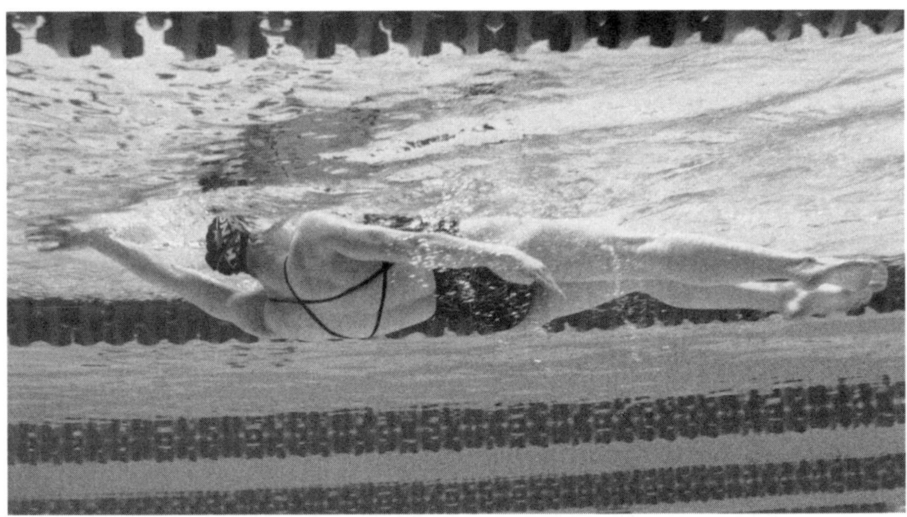

The finish is always done past the hips, fully extending the arm. Bringing the arm out of the water prior to that causes a big loss of power.

### Catch

"Grab" the water and begin to pull it at the top of your stroke. You can do this when you bend your arm close to a 90-degree angle and don't alter it, as it releases the water, until you finish your pull.

#### Olympian Tip Linking Each Stroke

***Adam Mania—***
***2004 Athens Olympian (Poland)***

It's best to be fluid when swimming backstroke and not to think about swimming one stroke at a time. Instead, link your strokes together. Each time you pause you have to start all over again, which takes additional energy, and it can be too easy to dip the hips if you stop moving.

# 5

# Butterfly

*Butterfly is the* most difficult stroke of the four to swim efficiently; that's not to say it's the most difficult to learn. Butterfly is actually a fairly simple stroke, merely one with a few facets that take a little more work to perfect. Whereas freestyle can be swum for miles on end with an inefficient form—as it sometimes is in pools around the world—butterfly, on the other hand, requires a greater grasp of technique in order to be swum for longer lengths.

Follow these steps and dedicate yourself to improving, and you'll be moving along in no time, much to the envy of everyone.

## BEGINNER'S BUTTERFLY

The easiest way to learn to swim butterfly is to begin training it in segments. Start training the kick, and learn the natural movement of the stroke. This will enable you to time the stroke properly and become a much more efficient swimmer.

Breaststroke and butterfly are both known as "short-axis" strokes due to their mechanics and undulation. One distinct difference, by numbers, is that in breaststroke you have one kick for every pull, whereas in butterfly you have two kicks for each pull (one small, one bigger).

### Kick

To start the kick, push off the wall underwater in the streamline position. Starting with the hips, whip your legs—feet together—and kick. Due to its similarities, the kick during this stroke is known

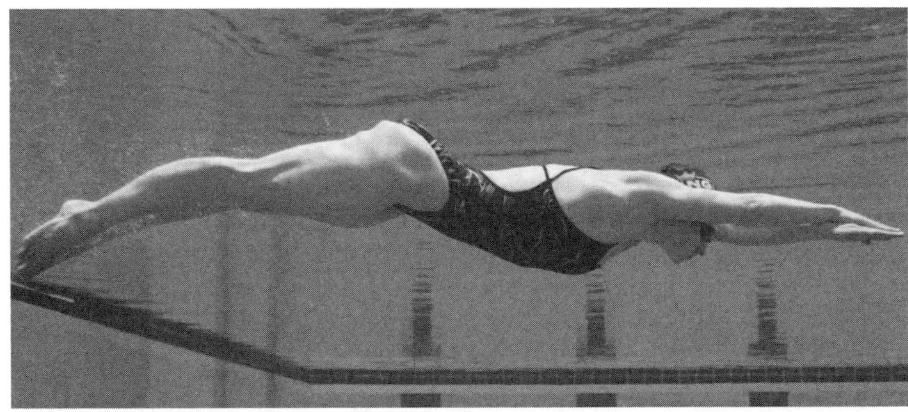

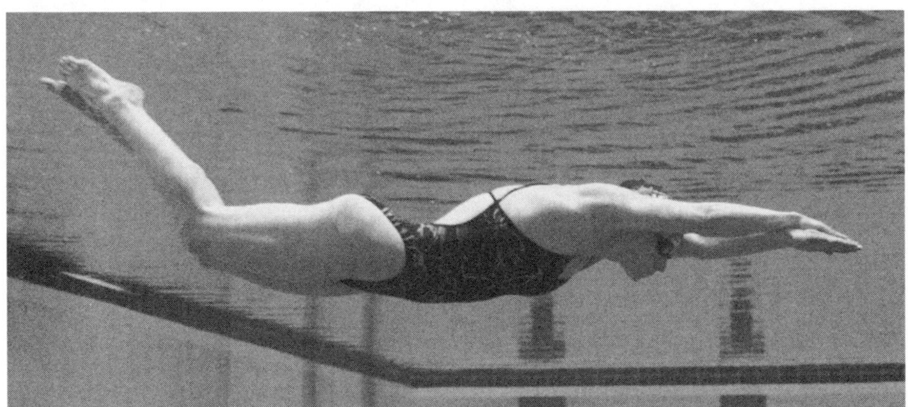

The dolphin kick is powered with the whole body, not just from the knees down. Use the hips to power the legs while maintaining a straight body position from the waist up.

as the "dolphin kick." Keep in mind that in competition it is illegal to use a flutter kick—kicking one leg at a time—doing butterfly. Even if you don't plan on competing, always practice proper technique.

### Pull

During butterfly your pull is timed against your kick. You begin your pull with your arms fully extended forward, entering the water in line with your shoulders, bending at the elbows and pulling back toward your hips. Make it a goal to enter your hands with as little splash as possible. Don't slap the water.

### Together

As your hands are entering the water, you proceed with your "big" kick downward. As you're pulling back and your hands are passing your hips, you add in a smaller kick.

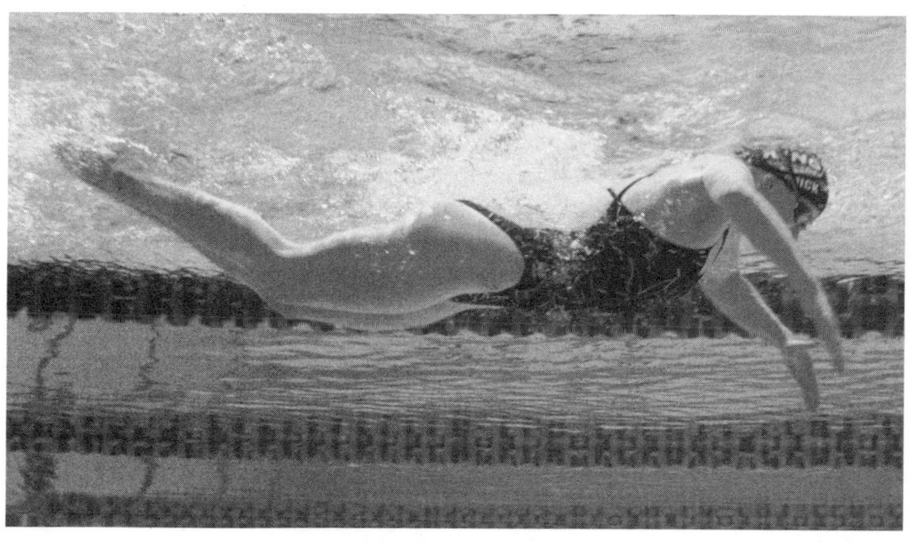

## Breathing

To breathe in butterfly, you lift your head as you're pulling your arms back past the hips. As your arms begin to come forward again, you drop your head back down into the water.

Don't give up on this stroke. It may take more practice, but that only makes it more rewarding when you make your stroke a thing of beauty to see.

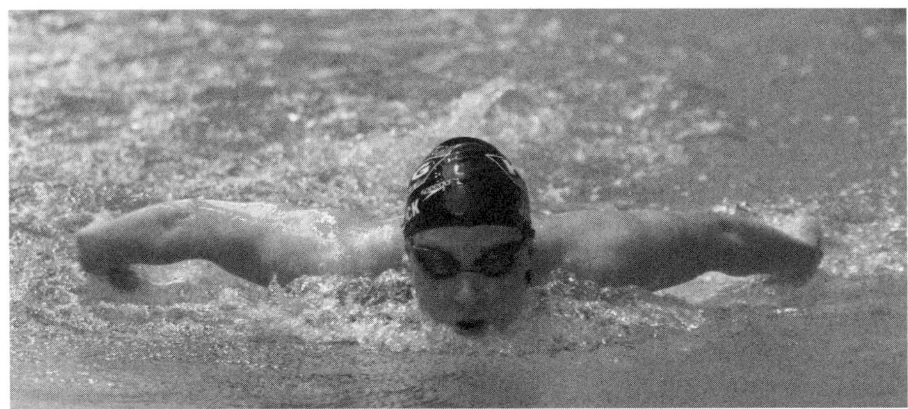

Because breathing in butterfly causes the hips to drop, lift your chin out of the water just enough to take in a quick breath, and return underwater to regain alignment. In learning stages people lift their head more than necessary to feel comfortable. Once you gain that comfort, work on lifting as little as possible.

## Common Mistakes to Avoid

First, you will definitely want to make sure that when you're recovering your arms over the water, they're relaxed. By keeping them tense and tight throughout the stroke, you will get tired much quicker. If you're able to get more comfortable and relaxed, you won't wear out as fast.

Next, be sure your breath is timed properly and directed correctly. Breathing is something that comes so naturally and is so mandatory that it's easy to assume you've got it down and not pay attention to it. Focus and be absolutely certain that what you're doing isn't putting your body out of line.

Finally, use your hips. They need to undulate enough to allow your body full range of motion and stretch into the stroke. If you're dragging your hips through the water, your stroke will be less effective, which will result in slower swimming and cause you to become fatigued much quicker.

## INTERMEDIATE BUTTERFLY

You now see how butterfly can be a pretty intricate stroke. As such, there are many technique changes you can make that will improve your speed and your ability to train for fitness with this stroke.

### Timing Your Air

This may be easier for some people at first than for others, but give it time and work, and you're sure to get it. In swimming fly, you're better off taking as few breaths as possible. That's because when you lift your head, your hips tend to drop, which increases drag and puts you out of the optimal alignment to swim.

Start with a one-up-one-down approach; that is to say, one stroke where your head stays underwater the whole cycle, followed by one with the head lifted, and keep repeating that.

### Head Position

Still on the breathing note, be sure you're not lifting your head too far when you come up for air. You'll know you're too far if you come up and see the other side of the pool. Ideally, you want to lift your head up and forward just enough to clear your mouth of the water and take in your breath. Your eyes should be at a downward angle on the water when your head is up.

### Hips

Your hips should be up toward the top of the water when your hands enter.

### Straight Arms

During the recovery phase of your stroke—which is when your hands are out of the water and preparing to enter again—keep your arms straight. It is easy to bend at the elbows during this part of the stroke, but it increases the likelihood that you'll be out of position. If you're riding too low in the water, where your hips are dragging you down, bending at the elbow is sometimes the only way to get your arms around. Keeping your arms straight will help keep you flat on top of the water, get you used to proper positioning, and provide you optimal hand-entry position.

## ADVANCED BUTTERFLY

Great Butterfly involves more than just a grip on the stroke. You need flexibility as well as strength, both attributes you will have developed better by the time you reach this point.

### Pressing

When recovering your arms, press your chest down. You will feel as if you're arching your back and keeping your hips up as your chest is down. This assists you in building and maintaining your stroke rhythm.

### Stretching

The larger the surface area of your pull, the better. If you look at Michael Phelps, for example, he reaches out as far as possible and bends enough that all portions of his arms that can effectively pull water are doing so at the earliest possible moment. Stretch out, grab the water, and pull.

Now that you can swim fluidly and are comfortable with stroke mechanics, you can begin shaping your body exactly as you have always wanted.

As you start training and adding more yardage and more varied swimming, you'll challenge your body in new and rewarding ways. Swimming helps build both body and mind, so challenge yourself and enjoy!

### Breathing Pattern

Few swimmers can get away with breathing too often if they want to really excel in butterfly, and those who do are exceptionally talented with years upon years of work in their craft. Still, you see the majority of the world's elite butterfly swimmers with a set breathing pattern. Try to do this when working on your stroke as well.

While ensuring that you bring your chin up the minimum amount to get air, try using the one-up-one-down pattern as covered in the Intermediate notes. Once you get used to that, try one-up-two-down. Depending on the length of your set, you may need to vary this pattern, but as previously mentioned, the fewer times you need to lift your head, the better.

6

# Starts

Even if as of right now you don't plan on ever competing in an actual swimming race, you'll want to learn how to properly start a race. Why? Because you never know if that competitive bug will hit you, and there's always an opportunity to gauge your progress. There are age-group meets all around the world, as well as a very strong Masters swimming organization (United States Masters Swimming) that is full of people who love the sport, support one another, and share a love of swimming.

Challenging yourself against the clock is great physically and mentally, especially when you envision yourself at the starting end of an Olympic pool.

If you're already a swimmer who enjoys racing in organized competition, look at these tips for starts and think critically about your own technique to make sure you're getting the most speed possible out of your fastest moments in the pool.

## FLAT START

There are two positions to start from. One is the "track" start, where the feet are staggered on the block; the other is the "flat" start, where both feet start at the edge of the block. The choice is yours, but we'll discuss the traditional flat start here first.

The flat or "grab" start begins with just your toes over the edge of the block, shoulder width apart, knees bent. Bend at the waist and grip the block. Keep your weight balanced over your feet, and don't lean back. Most of us have a natural tendency to lean back because it feels powerful, but if you do so, the first thing you have to do once the buzzer goes off is pass the same point you could have started at, which ultimately costs you time.

As you're leaving the block, push from the legs. Don't just fall into the water, give it some effort from the bottoms of your feet up through your core. Throw your arms forward rather than nonchalantly lifting them up. There should be nothing mundane about a start; starts should be powerful, explosive movements that, when racing, can be used to put you in the lead right from the start.

Go out, not up, as you're moving forward. Up is a slower path. Think of it like a football pass; a rainbow toss isn't nearly as fast as a straight bullet. You want to come off the block and go forward powerfully into a streamline.

When you enter the water, pretend there's a small ring on the surface. You want your whole body to go through this circle, starting with your fingertips. Enter at an angle and straighten your body so your whole self follows through this point. You want to enter rigid, like a broomstick, not bent at the elbows or the waist or the knees.

## TRACK START

For those interested in the track start, the same principles of entering in a straight, clean line apply. The differences here are your starting position on the blocks and the area where your force is derived.

With the track start, you'll place one leg forward in the same position as if it were a flat start. The other leg will be placed roughly twelve inches behind the heel of the other foot, but still in the same line as its flat-start positioning.

When you push off, use the force from both legs. It's easy to push with just one leg, but then you're not only losing out on force, you'll be dragging dead weight behind you. Start pushing with your rear leg, and as it begins moving forward, push as hard as you can with your opposite leg and, again, throw your arms out ahead of you to lead the charge into the water.

Expert Tip **Starts in Detail**

***Russell Mark—***
***USA Swimming Biomechanics Coordinator***

Even for an inexperienced spectator, it can be easy to tell who has a good start and who doesn't among a field of swimmers with varying start ability. When everyone pops up and starts swimming, if one swimmer already has a visible lead, it's evident that he or she has a great start. What makes a great starter so good? How can an average start become great? Certainly, a swimmer's underwater kicking ability is a factor, but if you look carefully you might be able to see that some swimmers appear to immediately surge ahead of everyone else after hitting the water. Even at the Olympic level, where every swimmer is among the best in the world, there are swimmers whose starts clearly stand out above the rest and provide a distinct advantage.

While most people are able to recognize the end result of a good start, the causes of a great start aren't as obvious. Without knowing the true roots of what makes or breaks a start, swimmers will find it hard to improve their start to make it the best possible. It's common for people to work on reaction time, distance off the blocks, or time to hit the water in order to improve their start, but while all of these are definite factors that impact the effectiveness of a start, there is only one factor that truly matters: forward velocity.

A great start is all about (1) generating forward velocity off the blocks, (2) how quickly a swimmer can generate that forward velocity from the start position, and (3) being able to maintain that forward velocity through the entry into the water.

In order to generate maximum forward velocity off the blocks, you need a great takeoff position. The takeoff position is not to be confused with the initial start position (which will be discussed later). It's the exact point when your legs are about to extend and push off the blocks, and at that point, they must be pushing your body forward. Focus on jumping forward instead of upward! That's the key. To do that, keep your upper body low throughout the transition from your initial start position to the takeoff position. *Prior* to pushing off the blocks with your legs, you want to have the sensation that your body is falling forward. If your body is leaning over the water and in front of the blocks, your legs will drive your body forward when they extend and push off. Think about generating forward velocity by jumping horizontally. The only way to jump horizontally is by having your body positioned in front of the blocks when your legs explosively push off the edge of the block.

It's true that your body travels much faster through air than through water, but while jumping upward creates a situation where a swimmer can maximize time (and therefore distance) in the air, the fact is that jumping upward doesn't maximize forward velocity, and that's what really matters.

When the start signal goes off, the natural instinct for most people is to throw their arms forward in order to get off the blocks as quickly as possible. The truth is that if the initial reaction is to forcefully throw with the arms, there is a tendency to lift the upper body too much and then jump in a direction that is too upward. If you are going to throw your arms after the start signal, just be careful of not "standing up" too much.

The most effective way to go from your initial start position to the best takeoff position is to use your arms to pull your body forward. This action is not to be confused with throwing your arms and upper body forward. With a firm grip on the edge of the block and the thumbs wrapped over the edge of it, pull your body toward your hands and you will tip your body forward to that ideal takeoff position. Obviously, the better the pull, the faster you'll get to the takeoff position and the quicker your start will be.

This is where the start position comes into play. One of the most common questions I hear is "What start position is better: a track start or a grab start?" There are pros and cons to both starts, but in recent years, the vast majority of world-class swimmers have been using a track start—where the feet are staggered with one foot at the front of the block and the other foot toward the rear of the block—including all of the best starters on the U.S. National Team. The main attraction of the track start is that most people feel it gives them a better reaction time off the blocks, but the true advantage of the track start is that it provides the most effective way to get from the initial start position to the takeoff. With the rear foot planted just behind the hips, the rear-leg push combines with the arm pull to move the body forward and generate forward velocity very quickly. Subsequently, the front leg pushes off the block with all of that momentum behind it. Some swimmers find that they are able to pull with their arms much more effectively when they are leaning back and "slingshot" themselves off the block, but this is not true for everyone and I believe that whether you are more comfortable with a front-weighted or rear-weighted track start depends on your body proportions, hamstring flexibility, and arm/leg strength ratio.

When performing a track start, it's important to keep in mind that your knees and toes should be pointing forward, since that's the direction you want to jump. A common mistake is for the back foot to be pointing out toward the side of the pool. Additionally, be certain that your feet are planted shoulder width apart, as if you were jumping normally on land.

Even though the grab start—with both feet starting at the front of the block—is currently going out of style in today's swimming world, it is still important to know about it so you can choose the best start position for yourself. The advantage of the grab start is that some people find it to be a more natural jumping position, and with a simultaneous push from both legs it can generate a greater jumping force. However, because there is no rear-leg push to help tip the body forward, the common initial movement from this start position is to throw the arms forward instead of pull with them. As stated earlier, throwing the arms can easily lead to a misdirected, upward jump.

The start definitely doesn't end with the takeoff and flight in the air. The entry is equally important, so that the swimmer can keep as much forward velocity as possible when hitting the water. Without a good entry, a great reaction and takeoff are pretty much negated. A great entry consists of a perfectly streamlined body from fingertips to toes—your head should be pressed tightly between your arms, and your legs should be stiff and straight with the toes pointed. Most important, you must enter the water with a tight core, so that your body doesn't break at the midsection upon impact. A large amount of force will act upon your body from the impact of entering the water at such a high velocity, and if you do not keep your body in a straight line, your body will bend and create drag.

In addition to influencing forward velocity, the takeoff is another aspect that affects the entry. Jumping forward will lead to the best possible entry. If a swimmer jumps in an upward direction off the blocks, (1) he or she will have to readjust body position in midair—which could be difficult—in order to line up the body and have a clean entry, and/or (2) he or she will enter the water at a steep angle because of the high start and will either have a deep dive or be forced to change directions very quickly underwater, which will cause a loss of speed.

7

# Turns

*While starts are* fun, turns are even more important because everyone—except long-course 50-freestylers—has to do them at one time or another. Every pool ends, so you'll want to know the fastest way to get turned around and back to swimming.

There are several turns you should know, and in competitive stances they're easily divided up. Freestyle and backstroke swimming allow a flip turn, while breaststroke and butterfly require what is called an open turn. Both have their place, both are simple to learn, and learning both will definitely benefit your aquatic achievements.

## FREESTYLE FLIP TURN

Turns for both freestyle and backstroke resemble simple somersaults. As you're coming into the wall, you roll forward and push off in a streamline position with your feet shoulder width apart. It's only slightly more complicated than it sounds, and with a little practice it won't take you long to develop a great turn. Play with it a bit, as your height and speed will determine when to somersault forward.

To win a sprint freestyle race, you definitely have to have great flip turns. To win three gold medals in sprint freestyle racing, you have to have some of the most amazing flip turns of all time. And wouldn't it be great to learn from someone like that?

To give you a more in-depth look at flip turns, we've acquired the assistance of one of the world's greatest sprinters (see the bottom of this page).

## BACKSTROKE FLIP TURN

You will follow the same tips as laid out for freestyle on the actual flipping portion of a backstroke turn, but you have a different setup before getting there.

As you're coming into the wall swimming backstroke, you will use the flags as your guide. Flags are universally set at fixed positions

Olympian Tip **Improving Your Flip Turns at Every Wall**

***Rowdy Gaines—***
***three-time gold medalist, 1984 Los Angeles Olympics; member of International Swimming Hall of Fame and U.S. Olympic Hall of Fame***

**1. Accelerate**
Never slow down going into the wall. One of the big mistakes young (and old) swimmers make is that, when they approach the wall, they begin to "measure" and their speed begins to decelerate. The more speed you have going into the turn, the more momentum you will have coming off it.

**2. Keep Your Head Down**

The best swimmers in the world never lift their head up at any point in their race, and that includes the turn. Jenny Thompson (four-time Olympian, eight gold medals) is a good example of this. When she arrives at a big competition and new pool, she practices going into her turn and making her initial flip looking at the cross on the bottom of the pool, not at the wall.

**3. Tuck Your Chin**

As you make your initial tumble, throw your chin to your chest. The head is very heavy. It's like a bowling ball sitting on top of your shoulders. The weight of the head can sometimes be a detriment during the stroke, but in this case, use that mass to your advantage by going into a nice tuck and "throwing" your chin to your chest.

**4. Feet Shoulder Width Apart**

Simple, yet many come over feet together as they somersault (bringing the weight of a lot of water on the back of their legs). Or their feet are too far apart. Visualize a standing broad jump coming off the wall with knees bent, but not too much.

**5. Bottom Arm First**

When coming off the wall, you should initially be on your back, quickly rotating to your side. Your first stroke—which, by the way, is the single most important stroke you take—should be taken with the arm facing the bottom of the pool. Anthony Ervin (gold and silver medalist, 2000 Sydney Olympics) might have done this better than anybody.

**6. Streamline**

The most important word in all of swimming, at least from a technical standpoint, is "streamline." It is impossible to swim faster than when you push off the wall. Why not take advantage of that by streamlining correctly, in three easy steps:

1. One hand on top of the other
2. Thumb clasped around your bottom hand
3. Biceps squeezed against the back of your ears

in all standard pools. Most swimmers will take three to four more strokes once they reach the flags before rolling over and flipping. After that number of strokes, when they turn over, they're in the same position they would be if they were swimming freestyle. Experiment with your approach to determine what works best for you.

Assuming your stroke count is three, once you get to the flags, take three more strokes and roll over to your stomach. As you're doing so, you're permitted in backstroke to take one freestyle pull during the continuous motion of the turn.

If your third stroke was with your left arm, begin turning as the arm is pulling down. Bring your right arm over the water as you're getting onto your stomach, and pull the water with a freestyle stroke as you're tucking your head and rolling into the turn.

As your feet are setting on the wall, get your arms into streamline as quickly and tightly as possible, and push off of the wall with a focus on keeping your body flat. If you're not in line, you'll be causing drag and your kick will be greatly slowed.

With backstroke turns, you can kick off the wall with either a flutter kick or dolphin kick while on your back. For some people the latter is quicker, but for new swimmers, we're going to suggest you stick with a flutter kick while you're learning the basics. The kicks off the wall are the same as during swimming, but done more powerfully underwater as you don't have to focus on stroke balance.

Go through these steps slowly, and be sure you're kicking throughout the entire process.

## BREASTSTROKE AND BUTTERFLY OPEN TURN

The turn for butterfly and breaststroke is the same. Both have the swimmer coming into the wall stretched out after a stroke. Your timing into the wall is something that practice will teach you, and you'll want to take advantage of it because taking a half stroke into the wall—where you touch, arms bent, before finishing your stroke—will slow you down and prevent a smooth transition.

As you come into the wall, don't lift your head. This causes immediate drag. Come into the wall fully extended and flat, touch the wall, and let your body fold into it. A funny, but fitting, example is of a crash-test car. The wall is immobile, and the car on contact folds into itself. That's what you want your body to do.

Your hands touch first, but be sure not to grab. Most pools have a gutter at water level, so it becomes easy to wrap your fingers around it and pull yourself close. You won't need to do that if you're swimming fast into the wall, just as it's suggested you do in freestyle. That remains constant: You always want to come into the wall fast. If you come into the turn quickly, you won't need to grab the wall because your momentum will be pushing you in.

As your body is going forward, keep your chin tucked down to your chest, bend at the knees, and pull your knees up together as if you're tucking them into your chest. If you're turning to your left, start coming off the wall by pulling your left elbow back and tucking it to your side. Put your feet on the wall; at this point you'll be turned completely sideways. Bring your right arm over your head as you're falling back under the water, get into streamline, and push off and onto your stomach.

At this point, depending on your stroke, you have what is called either a pull-out (for breaststroke) or a kick-out (for butterfly, freestyle, and backstroke).

## BREASTSTROKE PULL-OUT

After coming off the wall in a tight streamline, you will get into what is called the pull-out of the stroke. Separate your hands from each other and bring them out to just outside shoulder width apart.

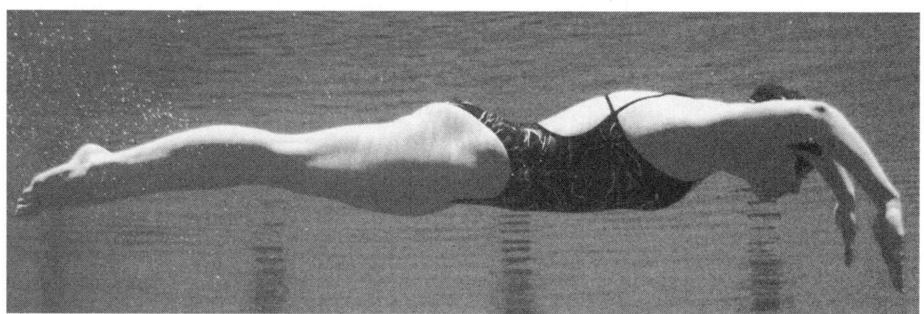

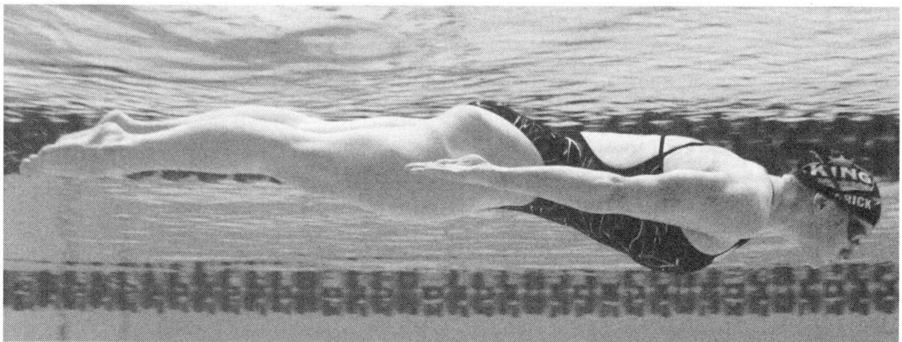

From streamline, move the arms apart and, similar to a butterfly pull, bend from the elbows down to gain as much surface area as possible for pulling water.

From here, bend down at the elbows and pull through to your hips (very similar to a butterfly pull).

At this point you'll be in something like a "torpedo" position with your hands at your hips and the rest of your body flat and straight. From here, you will slide your hands up underneath your stomach and chest on their way back out ahead of you. As they're passing your chest, you begin pulling your heels in, preparing for a kick.

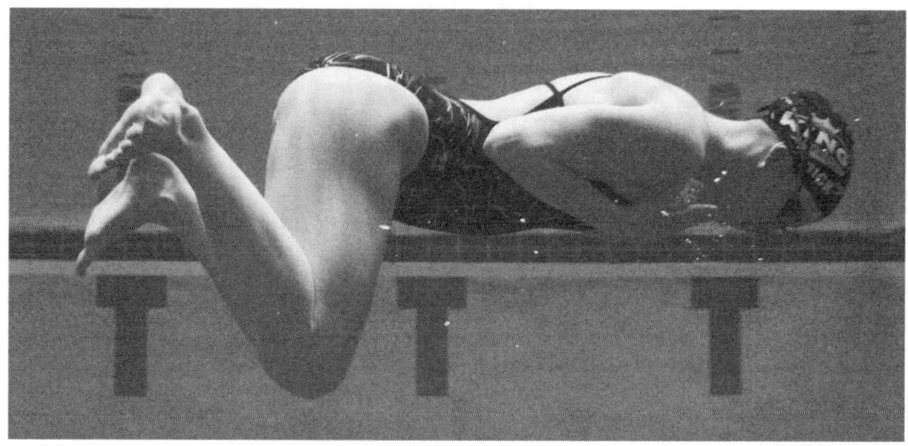

The hands slide up under the body as the legs go through the same motions as in a breaststroke kick. Pull the heels up to your bottom, point the toes out, and kick as the hands thrust forward.

As your hands pass your face, finish your kick and return to a flat position.

Your pull-out is now complete, and your next movement will be the beginning of a full stroke, which will also be the first time in the length you break the surface.

## BUTTERFLY KICK-OUT

Unlike in freestyle, where you're given the opportunity to choose a flutter or dolphin kick, in a butterfly race you have only the option of a dolphin kick. Keep a tight streamline and kick quickly and with as much force as possible. Once you begin to slow, break your streamline and start swimming.

8

# Racing Tips

This book has really focused on a lot of the things that we're commonly asked to elaborate on during the camps and clinics we headline. We'd like to continue that and cover something that is asked of Megan without fail at every clinic. That question is: "How do you get ready to race?" This will be more informative than instructional, but you may find some things here that you'd like to incorporate into your own preparation.

In the past, Megan has tried many methods of preparing for a race. Some people don't like to eat much before they swim, while others have to get a big meal in before the meet starts. Whereas some people warm up for only a few minutes, others take an hour. Some people stretch, some people don't. What's important to remember is, much like a training program or a nutritional program, the same thing won't work for every person.

For Megan, a day of competition always starts with a breakfast rich in protein and complex carbohydrates (nutrition is also covered elsewhere in this book). For her, a big breakfast has always been the best bet to ensure a steady stream of nutrients throughout the first hours of the day.

Preparation, too, is key. Everything has to be in order so that she can focus on racing. One way of making sure nothing will be forgotten is that she packs her swim bag the night before; suits, caps, goggles, towels, and snacks are all taken care of beforehand.

At the meet, Megan adopts a two-warm-up tactic that has her getting in the water and loosening up as soon as she arrives at the pool. During this first warm-up, she does the majority of her distance and she mixes in pulling, kicking, and medley swimming (all four strokes). Often, she'll use something like a parachute to provide some progressive resistance, which is to add drag to help develop power.

During her second warm-up, starting forty-five to fifty minutes before her race, Megan prepares with shorter repeats of swimming and introduces more short sprints into her routine.

When the second warm-up is complete, she dries off, switches into her racing suit, and concentrates on going as fast as possible when the time comes.

Behind the blocks, Megan stretches and waits patiently, focusing on putting into practice everything she has trained to do.

As mentioned earlier, some people choose not to stretch before their races, and this isn't actually a bad idea, though for many years it had gone against conventional wisdom. More and more research over the last few years has shown that static stretching before physical activity can decrease power and actually *increase* the chance of injury. One U.S. Army study published in the *Journal of Strength and Conditioning Research* found that a full-body warm-up is a superior choice. Some attendees of our clinics are followers of this type of research and ask why elite athletes still stretch in light of the studies.

The answer to this, which leads us back to different things working for different people, is that stretching is comfortable for a lot of people. Swimming in particular places high value on feeling "long" in the water, which is a feel that can be obtained by stretching the muscles. In addition, many athletes for one reason or another tend to cramp up during races, and this problem is often assisted by stretching out. Our advice is to try both methods before your next two races and see which is best for you.

After a race, many athletes can become discouraged based on their time. We urge you not to judge yourself based solely on the time on the clock.

Often swimmers will say, "I wasted that race," referring to the time they spent getting ready for a competition and then not performing up to their high standards. Ask yourself, "Did I learn something?" If you did, you didn't waste the race. In fact, you benefited from it. If you went out there but didn't learn anything, then you

Olympian Tip **Racing Wisdom from an Olympic Legend**

***Gary Hall Jr.—***
***ten-time medalist, 1996 Atlanta, 2000 Sydney, 2004 Athens Olympics***

Practice racing.

There is nothing that you can think of five minutes before your race that will have a positive impact. Just try to stay calm and focused. Avoid negative thoughts. Have faith in what you have been doing all season. This is the race you've been training for. Now just smile, flex your muscles for the crowd, and enjoy it. You've worked hard for those muscles, and you're about to swim a great race.

should reevaluate what you're doing. There should always be at least something, even if it's a small correction, that you realize after each race. Even the races you win should teach you something.

Everyone loses at some point or another. Megan, Michael Phelps, Brendan Hansen, Katie Hoff, and all of the other elite swimmers in the world all share something: Sometimes they lose. And it's okay, because they take something away from those races and it gives them the drive to keep training hard.

A motto hanging in our home reads, "You Can Always Better Your Best," and that's something that athletes should really focus on. Even after winning a gold medal or setting a world record, a swimmer should always be looking for ways to improve.

When you're racing, remember that you're not just racing the clock, you're also competing against yourself. If you went out there and felt that you made some of the changes you had recently been working on, even if it wasn't a best time, you were successful because you accomplished your goal.

No matter what happens in the pool, remember that you're doing it for the love of the sport and not just to stop the clock before anyone else. That comes in time, and it will come a lot quicker if you enjoy what you're doing and keep focusing on improvement.

9

# Tools of the Pool

There are various "tools" available for a swimmer to use during his/her training. Similar to the gear a football player wears, swimmers merely take advantage of their products in a different way. One distinct advantage is that swimmers don't have to wear pads or helmets all the time, just a suit and goggles will suffice—unless you're old-school and can even go without the goggles!

The equipment that swimmers use is often referred to as their toys. These are simple and fairly inexpensive, and if within your budget should be picked up after you're comfortable in the water to enable new possibilities for your training.

Here are some simple descriptions of these toys so you will know what you're buying and why it will help you.

## KICKBOARD

A kickboard can be a multipurpose toy. Its main use is that of allowing a swimmer to place his or her arms on it, keeping the head out of the water, in order to focus solely on the kick of a stroke. This is not used in kicking drills when on your back. Keep in mind that a kickboard should not be used by athletes who have shoulder injuries because the position—arms floating, hips down—adds stress.

A kickboard can also be used in a pinch as a pull buoy.

## PULL BUOY

A pull buoy is a foam device molded to fit above swimmers' knees and provide buoyancy when swimming, allowing the athlete to forgo use of his/her legs when swimming. Using a pull buoy, a swimmer can better focus on the pulling portion of his/her stroke. This is particularly beneficial when working on specific technique points in the pull, such as ensuring correct positioning.

One of the bigger problems new swimmers have is placing their hands properly during a pull because their hips tend to ride low in the water. When they don't have to worry about keeping their hips high because of the buoyancy of the buoy, they are able to concentrate on upper-body motion and learn the feel of a stroke with proper body positioning.

## PADDLES

Paddles give swimmers the feel of a stronger pull and teach proper positioning. A key benefit of using paddles is that if your hand is in the wrong position (such as cupped) the paddle will correct that merely by being flat. Using slower strokes, a swimmer can literally feel the changes of slight alterations during a pull. One example is that if swimmers are pulling directly back—a common problem among those who don't bend at the elbow—they will feel little resistance. When they correct this problem, they will feel a good amount of resistance as well as feel a strong pull through the water.

## FINS

Not necessarily a huge asset to advanced swim training, fins can offer a degree of comfort for the beginning swimmer. Wearing fins provides great buoyancy and balance in the water while assisting ankle flexibility. If you're uncomfortable getting going with a program, fins may be good for you; just be sure that you don't come to rely on them. If you are already confident in your swimming, fins can be used for some great leg-endurance sets because they increase the amount of water resistance against the leg.

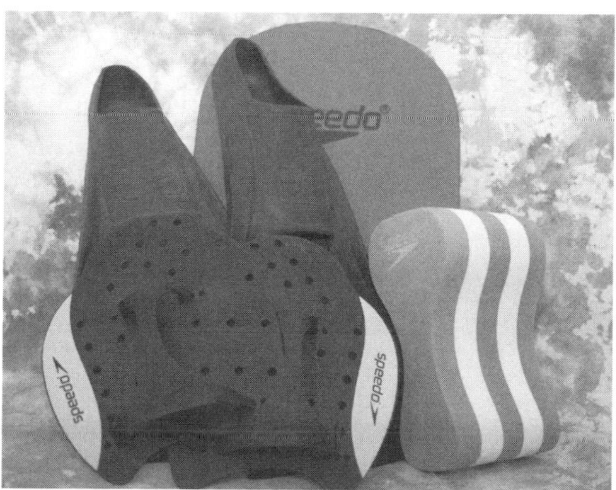


Shown here are fins, paddles, a pull buoy, and a kickboard. All are accessories that can enhance your training.

10

# Training Sets

This section of the book is dedicated to giving you actual workouts you can take to the pool and work through. They're divided up into different levels, from Beginner's to Advanced, starting very basic so that you can ease into swimming for fitness. Progressively they will add yardage and intensity to provide you a host of benefits.

Beginner's Sets will act as both a starting point for new swimmers and a refreshing point for older swimmers and individuals just getting back into the sport. This includes people who swam in high school or summer leagues, or just regular recreational swimmers.

Beginner's Sets will focus mainly on freestyle and backstroke swimming, with workouts emphasizing moderation and gaining comfort with the water.

Remember, when doing the workouts that follow, you don't have to go through them in order. If you like one, feel free to repeat it. Likewise, just because you've finished all of the Beginner's workouts, you don't have to move on to the Intermediate level if you're not prepared. Reuse workouts and mix and match to come up with some creative sets of your own.

## IMPORTANT NOTATIONS

You're going to see some notations in the following workouts that you may not have seen before. So here's a brief explanation of what you'll need to know.

**IM** stands for Individual Medley. You'll see it used as a set description, which means medley order: butterfly, backstroke, breaststroke, freestyle.

**Free/IM** is the same as IM, with the exception of changing out the initial butterfly for freestyle. So instead of going fly, back, breast, free, you'll be going free, back, breast, free.

**Over kick** means to kick as fast as possible while maintaining a normal stroke rate with the arms.

**Pull** means to use a pull buoy and use only the upper-body motion of the stroke.

**Kick** can be done with a kickboard or from the streamline position, lifting your head just enough to breathe when needed.

**Choice** means you can choose the pull/stroke/kick for the set noted.

**Length** refers to one length of the pool, typically twenty-five yards. Some pools in the United States and most pools abroad are twenty-five meters. Olympic-size pools are fifty meters.

## INTERPRETING A WORKOUT

### Example

2 x 25 butterfly @ :40

4 x 50 freestyle @ 1:00

2 x 100 Free/IM @ :20 seconds rest

For the workouts, the first number indicates how many of the following distance and stroke you will be doing. The example shows two repeats of 25 yards/meters of butterfly swimming on a forty-second send-off. That is to say, if you're looking at the pace clock and the second hand is on the 10, you should be leaving for the second swim on the 50. The second line of the example shows four 50-yard swims of freestyle, one leaving each minute. If you finish in forty-five seconds, you have fifteen seconds of rest before swimming again. The last line shows two times through a 100-yard swim of Free/IM, which is explained earlier, and in this case is broken out to one length freestyle, one backstroke, one breaststroke, and finally freestyle again. The notation for rest is twenty seconds of rest after each swim.

# BEGINNER'S SETS

## Beginner's Workout #1

Total yards: 300

4 x 25 freestyle

4 x 25 kick with a board choice

4 x 25 freestyle

Take as much rest as you need between lengths and sets, but try to be consistent in the length of each rest interval.

## Beginner's Workout #2

Total yards: 400

4 x 25 freestyle

2 x 50 kick with a board choice

4 x 25

Odd—freestyle

Even—backstroke

1 x 100 kick with a board choice

In this workout think about the amount of rest you took during Workout #1. Then try cutting about 10 seconds off. For example, if you were at about 2 minutes rest between each distance in Workout #1, then try for about 1:50 during this workout.

## Beginner's Workout #3

Total yards: 550

2 x 25 freestyle

2 x 50 freestyle

2 x 25 backstroke

2 x 50 backstroke

2 x 75 kick, resting as much as necessary between the two

100 your choice of stroke

If you were comfortable with the amount of rest in Workout #2, cut another 10 seconds of rest time off. This workout is also a great opportunity to put in some work on flip turns, given the length of the sets.

## Beginner's Workout #4

Total yards: 800

Starting with this workout, begin picking something to focus on each time you're in the water, such as not overreaching or making sure you're always steadily kicking as you swim.

4 x 50 alternate freestyle, backstroke by 50

2 x 100 kick with a board

4 x 75 alternate freestyle, backstroke by 50

4 x 25 freestyle pull with a pull buoy

Try to get your rest interval down to about 45 seconds after each distance and hold it at :45 or better for the remainder of the workout.

## Beginner's Workout #5

Total yards: 800

2 x 100 freestyle

1 x 200 kick with a board choice

4 x 25 IM (1 of each stroke)

4 x 50 pull with a pull buoy freestyle

4 x 25 @ 2:00 freestyle or backstroke fast. Be sure you're not sacrificing your technique for speed.

## Beginner's Workout #6

Total yards: 850

This workout introduces you to longer, 200-yard continuous swims. Keep in mind that these may be difficult, but they're here with the intent of developing your endurance base.

1 x 200 freestyle

1 x 200 backstroke

1 x 200 your choice of stroke kick with a board

2 x 100 pull with a pull buoy freestyle

1 x 50 your choice of stroke fast

## Beginner's Workout #7

Total yardage depends on your long swim amount

Do the entire workout with fins. This will make swimming a little easier and allow you to focus on your technique.

1 x 300 alternate freestyle, backstroke by 50

3 x 100 kick on your back. You're not using a board, so you need to float. Remember to keep your hips and feet near the surface of the water. A trick for doing that is pulling your head back and tightening your abs a bit.

*Long swim.* Wearing your fins, swim as many laps as you can without stopping. Before you do this, set a goal of how many you would like to do. If the alternating 300 earlier felt smooth, try to aim now for at least 16 lengths (400 yards).

## Beginner's Workout #8

Total yards: 1,000

With this workout, pick a specific technique during each set that you may be having trouble with and focus on fixing it and swimming properly.

200 freestyle or backstroke

8 x 25 IM (2 of each stroke)

12 x 25 @ :20 seconds rest your choice of stroke

Odd—fast

Even—focusing on technique

1 x 200 kick on your back with fins

2 x 50 pull with a pull buoy freestyle

## Beginner's Workout #9

Total yardage depends on your long swim amount.

2 x 150 alternate freestyle, backstroke by 50

2 x 100 kick on your back (hips and feet near the surface)

2 x 50 pull with a pull buoy freestyle

*Long swim*. This time freestyle without fins. Again, set a goal amount and see if you can reach it!

### Beginner's Workout #10

Total yards: 1,100

1 x 400 freestyle or backstroke with fins

12 x 25 IM (3 of each stroke)

1 x 200 kick on your back freestyle

4 x 25 breaststroke kick with a board

4 x 25 IM fast

### Olympian Tip Beating Bad Days in the Pool

***Scott Goldblatt—silver medalist, 2000 Sydney Olympics, gold medalist, 2004 Athens Olympics***

Everyone has good days and bad days in the pool. Olympians are no different—we are human, and I, for one, have had a lot of bad days. I always tried, but often the level of performance I expected just was not there. But when it was not there, I instead made a specific focus on my swimming. I may have been going slowly, I may have been tired, I may have been missing intervals, but I never gave up and never lost focus on my stroke. If I was not going to make intervals, I never just stopped. I swam straight through the set with a focus on each and every stroke. I focused on my high elbows during my recovery, on rotating my hips and getting the most length out of every stroke, and on every underwater pull.

It is not overstated to focus on every stroke. It helped me and gave me the opportunity to improve—a couple thousand times a day.

# INTERMEDIATE SETS

Welcome to the next level of swimming workouts. If you've become comfortable with the Beginner lessons, you're already an accomplished individual who has a solid grasp on a life-changing skill. You should be noticing enhanced muscle mass, flexibility, and a high level of confidence with your skills.

Before you start this next level of training, keep in mind that not everyone progresses at the same rate. If you find these workouts a little uncomfortable in the sense that you're not quite making the send-offs, don't be afraid to revisit the prior workouts. Even better, once you've completed all of them you can mix and match and really take charge of your training by designing your own workouts. On any of these workouts, if you're moving smoothly but just aren't quite fast enough, go ahead and adjust the rest period or goal time for the set. This is your program, adjust it to fit; the times we have included are just guidelines to help.

## Intermediate Workout #1

Total time: Approximately 1 hour

Total yards: 2,050

### Warm-up

200 freestyle

100 IM

4 x 50 kick @ 1:20

**2 rounds through warmup**

### Main Set

12 x 50 @ 1:15 alternate freestyle, backstroke by 25. See if you can kick out at least 5 yards, or to the flags, each time you push off the wall

8 x 25 @ :55 your best stroke focusing on technique

### Cooldown

5 x 50 alternate freestyle, backstroke by 25

## Intermediate Workout #2

Total time: Approximately 1 hour

Total yards: Approximately 1,950

### Warm-up

3 x 150 freestyle @ 2:30, 2:20, 2:10

200 IM pull with a pull buoy

2 x 75 @ 1:30 kick

2 x 25 @ :40 your choice of stroke 15 meters fast

### Main Set

Take about 10 minutes and start working on your kick-outs. Try doing a few 25's fly kick on your back, making sure that you kick out underwater at least past the flags each time.

4 x 25 @ 1:00 fast your choice of stroke fast focusing on kick-outs/ pull-outs

1 x 50 @ 1:30 easy any stroke

**4 rounds**

### Cooldown

4 x 100 your choice of stroke

## Intermediate Workout #3

Total time: Approximately 1 hour

Total yards: 1,850

### Warm-up

300 alternate stroke by 50

100 kick

100 pull

### Main set

200 pull your best stroke

100 pull your best stroke

50 pull your best stroke

**3 rounds through main set**

Take as much rest as you need between each of these. Focus on a specific technique for the stroke you are doing. When Megan works on breaststroke pulling, for example, she focuses on grabbing as much water as possible and accelerating with each pull. She makes sure that her elbows don't go too far back behind her shoulders.

### Cooldown

3 x 100

- 1st—pull
- 2nd—kick
- 3rd—swim freestyle

## Intermediate Workout #4

Total time: Approximately 1 hour

Total yards: 2,050

### Warm-up

2 x 200

1st—freestyle

2nd—backstroke

200 free/IM pull (entire 200 is pull; free/IM indicates doing IM but doing freestyle instead of fly)

4 x 50 kick

### Main Set

8 x 50 @ 3:00 your choice of stroke as fast as possible. Even though these are fast, make sure you are focusing on your technique as well.

400 easy freestyle

8 x 25 @ 1:00 your choice of stroke fast, focusing on technique

### Cooldown

10 x 25 @ :40 focusing on technique, your choice of stroke

## Intermediate Workout #5

Total time: Approximately 1 hour

Total yards: 2,250

### Warm-up

300 alternate by 50, your choice of stroke

200 pull

100 kick

### Main Set

6 x 100 @ :30 rest freestyle. The focus on this should be on your kick. Try working on the technique of your kick as well as taking more kicks for each stroke cycle.

1 x 50 @ :45

1 x 100 @ 1:35 freestyle with fins. These send-offs may be fast for some people. This is intended to get your heart rate up with very little rest in between so it stays elevated.

**3 rounds**

### Cooldown

300 alternate by 50

200 pull freestyle

100 kick your choice of stroke

## Intermediate Workout #6

Total time: Approximately 1 hour

Total yards: 2,400

### Warm-up

5 x 150 @ :30 rest

1st—swim freestyle

2nd—pull

3rd—kick

4th—swim freestyle with paddles

5th—swim freestyle

### Main Set

10 x 25 @ 1:10 butterfly kick on your back underwater. Try to do this without any breaths. This will be fairly hard, so if you do need a breath, come up to the surface, get a breath, and return to the fly kick underwater as quickly as possible. Also be sure you're starting your kick at your hips, not just from your knees.

8 x 150

2 freestyle

2 your best stroke pull with a pull buoy

2 freestyle

2 your best stroke pull with a pull buoy

### Cooldown

4 x 50 alternate freestyle, backstroke by 25

## Intermediate Workout #7

Total time: Approximately 1 hour

Total yards: 2,500

### Warm-up

5 x 100 @ :10 rest your choice of stroke

200 kick

### Main Set

100 @ :15 rest freestyle

4 x 25 @ :40 your best stroke pull

100 @ :15 rest your choice of stroke

4 x 25 @ :40 your best stroke

On the 100s, focus on getting faster throughout the 100, with each length getting progressively more effort put into it. On the 25s, focus on your best pulling and swimming technique, keeping in mind something specific for each length.

**3 rounds**

### Cooldown

2 x 300 alternate freestyle, backstroke by 50

## Intermediate Workout #8

Total time: Approximately 1 hour

Total yards: 3,500

### Warm-up

300 alternate by 50 your choice of stroke

4 x 75 @ :10 rest kick

300 free/IM pull

### Main Set

400 free/IM

400 freestyle

200 free/IM

200 freestyle

Take 20 seconds rest after each set. The focus should be on turns, kick-outs, and stroke technique. This is to help build your endurance, so you don't want your heart rate above 70% of maximum.

**2 rounds**

### Cooldown

200 easy your choice of stroke

## Intermediate Workout #9

Total time: Approximately 1 hour

Total yards: 2,600

### Warm-up

500 alternate by 50 your choice of stroke

4 x 75 @ :10 rest kick

300 your choice of stroke pull

### Main Set

4 x 50 @ 2:30 IM fast. The focus should be on good technique while still going fast.

200 easy freestyle

**2 rounds**

4 x 100 @ 1:55 freestyle with paddles fastest average. Go the fastest time you can hold for all the 100s.

### Cooldown

300 easy your choice of stroke

## Intermediate Workout #10

Total time: Approximately 1 hour

Total yards: 3,400

### Warm-up

4 x 150 fly, free, back, free, breast, free x 25 @ :20

1 x 200 kick

8 x 25 @ :45 your choice of stroke pull

### Main Set

12 x 150 @ :30 rest

- 4 freestyle, getting faster with each 150
- 4 your best stroke pull, focusing on technique
- 4 alternating butterfly, backstroke, freestyle, breaststroke, freestyle by 25

### Cooldown

6 x 100 @ :15 rest freestyle backstroke by 25

## ADVANCED SETS

These workouts should be attempted once you are very comfortable with the previous examples and when your technique feels solid.

### Advanced Workout #1

Total time: Approximately 1½ hours

Total yards: 4,000

#### Warm-up

4 x 150 @ 2:00 alternate freestyle, backstroke by 25

200 @ 2:50 IM pull

4 x 50 @ :50 kick with a board

1 x 25 fast freestyle

**2 rounds**

#### Main Set

1 x 150 @ 1:55 freestyle

2 x 75 @ :50 your best stroke

1 x 150 @ 1:50 freestyle

2 x 75 @ :55 your best stroke

1 x 150 @ 1:45 freestyle

2 x 75 @ 1:00 your best stroke

1 x 150 @ 1:40 freestyle

2 x 75 @ 1:05 your best stroke

1 x 150 @ 1:35 freestyle

2 x 75 @ 1:10 your best stroke

1 x 150 @ 1:30 freestyle

### Cooldown

6 x 50 @ :55 alternate freestyle, backstroke by 25

## Advanced Workout #2

Total time: Approximately 1½ hours

Total yards: 4,000

### Warm-up

3 x 300 @ 4:00, 3:40, 3:20 freestyle

400 @ 5:40 IM pull

4 x 75 @ 1:10 kick

2 x 50 @ 1:15 15 meters your choice of stroke fast

12 x 25 @ :55 butterfly kick on your back underwater. The focus on this is on kick-outs. Make sure you are doing this as fast as possible.

### Main Set

2 x 50 @ 2:00 your best stroke fast. Although this set is fast, the focus should be on turns, kick-outs, and pull-outs.

1 x 100 @ 2:00 easy your choice of stroke

**5 rounds**

### Cooldown

10 x 100 @ 1:45 IM focusing on turns and kick-outs

## Advanced Workout #3

Total time: Approximately 1½ hours

Total yard: 3,800

### Warm-up

600 alternate by 50 your choice of stroke

200 kick

200 pull

### Main Set

300 @ :30 rest your best stroke pull

200 @ :20 rest your best stroke pull

100 @ :10 rest your best stroke pull

This should be in your best stroke unless you have multiple "best strokes," in which case you can change by round. Pick a specific aspect of your pull to work on for this set, such as entry, elbow position, or finish.

**4 rounds**

### Cooldown

4 x 100 @ 1:40 alternate freestyle, backstroke by 25

## Advanced Workout #4

Total time: Approximately 1½ hours

Total yards: 2,800

### Warm-up

2 x 200 @ 2:40

1 x 400 IM pull

4 x 50 @ :55 kick

### Main Set

12 x 50 @ :55. The focus of this is on IM transition turns and kick-outs.

1st—alternate butterfly, backstroke by 25

2nd—alternate backstroke, breaststroke by 25

3rd— alternate breaststroke, freestyle by 25

Repeat ten times

4 x 100 @ 5:00

50 your best stroke fast

50 stroke following your best in IM order fast. Example: Best stroke is breaststroke= 50 breaststroke, 50 freestyle.

Do about 200 easy during your rest time after each 100.

4 x 50 @ 2:00

25 your best stroke fast

25 stroke following your best in IM order fast

4 x 25 @ 1:00 your best stroke as fast as possible

### Cooldown

500 easy your choice of stroke

## Advanced Workout #5

Total time: Approximately 1½ hours

Total yards: 4,100

### Warm-up

300 alternate by 50 your choice of stroke

200 pull

100 kick

**2 rounds**

### Main Set

12 x 50 @ 1:00 freestyle overkick—meaning kick as fast as possible. On the "overkick," take many more kicks with each stroke than you normally would. Your legs should be very tired at the end of each 50.

1 x 50 @ :35 freestyle with fins

1 x 100 @ 1:20 freestyle with fins

**6 rounds**

12 x 50 @ 1:15 kick fastest average. Go the fastest time you can hold for all the 50s.

### Cooldown

8 x 100 alternate freestyle, backstroke by 50

## Advanced Workout #6

Total time: Approximately 1½ hours

Total yards: 4,500

### Warm-up

5 x 300 @ :15 rest

1st—freestyle

2nd—pull

3rd—kick

4th—freestyle with paddles

5th—freestyle

### Main Set

12 x 25 @ :55 butterfly kick on your back underwater fast no breath

16 x 150 @ :20 rest

4 freestyle

4 your best stroke pull

4 freestyle

4 your best stroke pull

### Cooldown

300 your choice of stroke easy

## Advanced Workout #7

Total time: Approximately 1½ hours

Total yards: 3,600

### Warm-up

3 x 100 @ 1:30 freestyle

3 x 100 @ 1:20 freestyle

200 IM pull

4 x 50 @ :55 kick

8 x 25 @ :50 your best stroke kick underwater, no breath

### Main Set

1 x 150 @ 1:50 freestyle

4 x 25 @ :30 your best stroke pull

1 x 150 @ 1:40 freestyle

4 x 25 @ :30 your best stroke

**4 rounds**

On the free you should focus on descending or getting faster during the 150. On the 25s stroke you should be focusing on perfect technique.

### Cooldown

400 easy your choice of stroke

## Advanced Workout #8

Total time: Approximately 2 hours

Total yards: 5,600

### Warm-up

400 freestyle IM

200 backstroke pull

4 x 75 @ 1:25 kick

4 x 25 @ :30 your best stroke focusing on technique

**2 rounds**

12 x 25 @ :50

Odd—butterfly kick on your back fast

Even—Your best stroke fifteen meters, fast

### Main Set

3 x 75 @ 1:30 your best stroke

200 easy your choice of stroke

2 x 75 @ 1:45 your best stroke

200 easy your choice of stroke

1 x 75 @ 2:00 your best stroke

200 easy your choice of stroke

**2 rounds**

The 75s are in your best stroke. They should be at ⅓ of your best 200 LCM (Long Course Meters) time if you have one. For example, if you go a 2:09 200-meter freestyle, your pace on the 75s should be :43.

8 x 100 @ 1:30 freestyle pull with paddles fastest average. Go the fastest time you think you can hold on all the 100s.

### Cooldown

4 x 100 @ 1:25 alternate freestyle, backstroke by 25

## Advanced Workout #9

Total time: Approximately 2 hours

Total yards: 6,500

### Warm-up

400 alternate by 50 your choice of stroke

300 freestyle, IM pull

200 kick

4 x 50 @ 1:15

25 kick

25 swim fast your choice of stroke

**2 rounds**

10 x 100 @ 1:20 your choice of stroke (preferably freestyle or backstroke)

### Main Set

3 x 300 @ 3:40 freestyle. Build each 300:

1st—fast

2nd—faster

3rd—fastest

3 x 300 @ 4:15 freestyle, IM. Build each 300 same as above.

### Pull

5 x 200 @ :20 your best stroke pull. Make sure that after the main set, when you are tired, you are really focusing on your technique.

### Cooldown

500 alternate freestyle, backstroke by 50

## Advanced Workout #10

Total time: Approximately 2 hours

Total yards: 5,350

### Warm-up

1 x 300 @ 3:40 freestyle

100 your best stroke pull

200 kick

**3 rounds**

12 x 25 @ :45 your best stroke

1st—½ fast, ½ easy

2nd—½ easy, ½ fast

3rd—all easy

4th—all fast

**3 rounds**

### Main Set

1 x 150 fast from the blocks. The goal on this should be to be on pace for your best 200-yard time. For example, if your best 200-yard backstroke is a 2:08, you would want to be about a 1:36 for 150 yards.

500 your choice of stroke easy

**5 rounds**

### Cooldown

6 x 100 @ 1:40 freestyle focusing on your kick

If you've gone through some of the preceding Advanced workouts, congratulations! You've completed workouts similar to those created and done by an Olympian. You have an idea of the variety you can provide yourself in future workouts and a base of examples to work with.

If you want more prewritten sets, additional workouts for endurance, sprinting, and lactate threshold training can be found in the Cross-Training chapter later in this book.

# 11

# Drills

*As you've probably* guessed, there is more to swimming than just doing laps. Sure, you're always moving, but you need to make sure you're moving with a purpose. If you've followed everything we've said so far, you're getting a great workout. That's your purpose for putting in the effort. While this book isn't strictly about making you a faster swimmer—there's other good information out there on that, and we're focusing on getting you in the best shape of your life—everyone should share the goal of becoming more efficient. Without efficiency, you won't be able to train long enough in the water to complete your workouts because fatigue will set in too early.

There are countless drills you can do in the pool to help improve your feel for the water. Feel is something you have to gain before becoming an efficient swimmer; being tense in the water prevents you from getting the most out of your swimming. These drills, easy on the body and relatively simple to perform, will help you gain confidence in your abilities and allow you to take your fitness swimming to a higher level. The drills are also workouts themselves.

Drills also allow you a stress-free time to plug the holes in your technique. When doing a drill, you're able to focus on what you're doing, why you're doing it, and how to make it better. Often these drills—done at times by separating the upper- and lower-body movements—will reiterate to you how something should be done. Once you've had such an epiphany—(and some things will definitely seem like such)—you can go back to your strokes and they may very well feel completely different, in a very good way.

## SCULLING

Sculling is a very simple and very beneficial way to enhance your feel for the water. Essentially, you're using your arms as oars and pushing the water. The name, naturally, is derived from the rowing sport of sculling. These drills simply make your arms the oars and your body the boat.

Start by standing in water that is comfortably deep for you. Chest height is a great starting point. Put your arms out in front of you on top of the water, and flatten your hands while keeping your fingers together. Turn your hands so that your palms are facing out, and slowly push your hands out a few feet. Then turn your palms back to face each other and scull back toward the middle.

By doing this you're literally teaching yourself how water works and learning the "feel" that you search for when swimming any stroke. The goal in swimming is to pull as much water as efficiently as possible; to do that, you have to know where to push the water from. This teaches you the right surface area for best propulsion.

After you scull while standing a bit, try floating on your back and sculling in small figure eights with your hands down by your hips. You'll quickly find that you can easily move up and down the pool with this, which is a healthy drill for gaining comfort in the water as well.

## BACKSTROKE DRILLS

### Catch Rotation

On your back, with a steady flutter kick, hold one arm perpendicular in the water (pointing up toward the ceiling or sky). Pull with the other arm, and when that arm reaches your perpendicular one, switch. Leave the arm you just took a stroke with pointing upward, and take a stroke with your other arm. You should be focusing on body rotation with this drill.

### Nonrotation Drill

When some people swim backstroke, their body and head rotate too much and they end up "wiggling" their way down the pool and zigzagging throughout the lane. These are the types of people who in a 100-yard race may end up swimming 105 yards or so just because they move from side to side so much. This drill will help you to keep your body in a more straight, streamline position.

Take a water-bottle top and place it on your forehead when you are in the backstroke position. Then try to swim a length of backstroke keeping the bottle top in the same place on your forehead. If it falls off into the water, you are rotating your head and/or body too much.

## BREASTSTROKE DRILLS

### Two Kicks/One Pull

This drill is done by taking one full breastroke pull but extending the glide and adding a kick. After you finish your stroke and are back in the streamline position, continue underwater and kick again. As you approach the surface following the second kick, complete another full stroke. This can help you get higher in the water as well as make it easier to feel the acceleration of the stroke with your arms.

### Streamline Kick on Back

From the backstroke streamline position (so you're staring at the ceiling or sky), rather than flutter kick, go through the breaststroke motions. Focus on keeping your knees beneath the surface of the

Olympian Tip **Building a Kicking Base**

***Tommy Hannan—***
***gold medalist, 2000 Sydney Olympics***

Young swimmers need to think of themselves as a boat. The power and speed is generated in the rear, or at the engines. Your engines are your legs. Whether you are a world-class sprinter or a distance swimmer, having power to propel you comes from your engines. To build speed and endurance, start at the bottom and build up. If you build a strong foundation of kicking, everything else will fall into place.

water. This will improve the motion of how you want your kick to be when you're doing the actual breastroke swimming. If your knees break the surface, you'll know you're bringing more of your body out of line than you should, thus causing more drag.

When actually swimming breaststroke, you don't want to bend any more than necessary to get into the kicking position, as doing so will only slow you down.

## BUTTERFLY DRILLS

### Streamline Kick on Back

Take the streamline position on your back. This time, use a dolphin kick to propel yourself down the pool. This allows comfort by giving you freedom to breathe, and will allow concentration on your kicking motion.

If you have trouble doing this for long periods, one way to keep moving and still gain the benefits of this drill is to kick as far as possible off each wall with the drill, then swim backstroke to the end of the length. After you turn, start the next length with the original drill. Make it a goal to kick farther each time. This drill will also slightly work out your abs while increasing kick proficiency and body line.

### Three Kicks/One Pull

Streamline off a wall and do an underwater kick-out. Take one stroke and a breath, but after your recovery don't go right into your next stroke. After the hands return out in front of you, instead of pulling, return to streamline. Do three kicks underwater, and then take a breath as you add a pull. Repeat that pattern. Doing this will help you get a feel for a fluid kick in the water.

### One-arm Butterfly

This drill works with either arm but should be alternated to maintain a balance. To assist in your learning of the timing butterfly swimming requires, streamline off of each wall and begin swimming with only one arm. Leave the other arm straight and leading forward. Instead of breathing up, breathe to the side of the arm you are pulling with. Make sure you're focusing on the kick timing and finishing your hand all the way back past your hips. Swimming with one arm at a time allows you to focus on specific techniques.

### Arm Entry

Kick using a dolphin kick on the surface of the water with your arms out in front of you, bent at the elbows, with your shoulders at a 90-degree angle to the body. This is the position your arms should be in as you are pulling them back through the water. This drill will help you feel the water as you move through it and allow you to find this position easily when swimming the stroke.

## FREESTYLE DRILLS

### Catch-up

Swim with one arm always remaining in the streamline position out ahead of you. After coming off of each wall and breaking the surface, pull with one arm while leaving the other out until the pulling arm returns to meet it. Then pull with the other arm, and

12

# The Swimmer's Nutrition Program

Some of the best swim coaches in the United States believe that the recent rash of world record–breaking performances was caused not as much by advances in technique as it was by advances in nutrition. Every record that is broken is captured by an athlete who has properly fueled his or her body to perform at its optimal level. And while your personal goals may not include a world record, the objective stays the same: top personal performance.

Like anything, a proper nutrition program takes work. If it were easy, the majority of Americans wouldn't have weight problems. Unfortunately, due to an addictive eating nature we as a people are accustomed to, and to a great degree the additives in much of our processed foods, we are constantly taking in more and more calories and often we're not even aware of it. As certain documentaries (*Super Size Me*, for example) that have come out over recent years have suggested, portion sizes of food continue to grow while the energy requirements of people do not. The extra, of course, is stored as adipose tissue, which is more commonly known as no one's friend, "body fat." In addition, depending on their source, excess calories can lead to a host of unfriendly side effects that at the very least will prevent you from feeling your best.

One thing that most people are well aware of is that there is a host of diet programs out there, all boasting a load of promises but delivering very little in the way of results. When looking for a new structure for your everyday eating, don't look to a diet. We have all seen the fads come and go—Atkins, South Beach, Jenny Craig, and countless others—and they seem to work for some while failing many others. There's a reason for this: Most of these programs are not fitted to each individual's needs. As different as people are on the outside, we are just as different on the inside. People have different metabolisms. People have different levels of insulin sensitivity—that is, how they respond to sugar. People, in general, have different eating habits. Because of this myriad of reasons, and no doubt many more, one diet isn't going to work for everyone. You have to find a program—not a diet—that will work with your body and, to a good extent, your mind.

## PROPER EATING

As you've seen throughout this book already, and will see shortly, there are a number of different methods to train your body when it comes to swimming. Then there are the additives, which are very important, such as stretching and drills, and even further there's the dryland training. All of these things can complement one another, depending on the route you wish to take in achieving your physical fitness goals. Likewise, there's a similar approach when planning out your new eating habits. As with your training, you make it a lifestyle change, not a temporary adjustment. And there are several ways to reach your goals.

People look at diets as something they do for a while until they reach their desired appearance, and then often they change course and go back to eating as they did when they realized they needed to lose weight in the first place. Eventually, usually sooner than expected, they are back where they had originally started, and the only things they're left with are a great deal of wasted time, dashed expectations, and a good amount of disappointment. In addition, research has found that yo-yo dieting, as constant weight loss followed by weight gain is called, can cause people to gain pounds more easily in later years.

But this can all be avoided by not going on a diet in the first place.

Proper eating, especially when fueling an athletic body, is a lifestyle decision and not a brief stint of visiting your local health food store. While permanently changing dietary habits may sound difficult to some people, it's really very simple and it doesn't take nearly as much work as it seems. In fact, it's a gradual process that leaves you not just satisfied, but with results you can see and maintain for life. Many people are shocked at how their life changes from an everyday perspective when they adjust the foods they consume on a daily basis. They feel more energetic and more refreshed each morning, recover more quickly, have increased self-esteem, and just enjoy their lives more. It's a feeling not reserved for those in Hollywood or those who can afford pricey home-gym equipment advertised on late-night infomercials; it's there for the taking, for everyone.

As we begin, there are a few things to keep in mind:

1. Proper nutrition is not a temporary alteration of your daily diet. If you revert to your old habits, you'll both look and feel as you did before. As is often said, if you do the same things, you'll only get the same things.

2. There is no such thing as a magic pill for weight loss. In fact, many thermogenic fat-loss aids can actually be counterproductive (which we will cover soon). The Swimmer's Nutrition Program is as natural as the foods you choose to eat—no expensive, overmarketed pills required. While there are many vitamin and mineral supplements that can enhance your health, absolutely zero is required to achieve your goals.

3. Results are gradual and patience is required. The adage "If it seems too good to be true, it probably is" may very well apply to dieting more than anything else. We'll debunk some myths next, and you'll see what we mean.

## DIET MYTHS

There is a load of promises being marketed to the world when it comes to diet pills, special drinks, "celebrity secrets," and more. They're all based around health and beauty because there's so much value placed on these attributes. We want you to feel blessed to be who you are, and feel blessed that you're in your own skin. You have control over your own body, and whatever your goals are, you can and will achieve them if you try hard enough. Hollywood isn't always reality, which is certainly something to remember.

One of the most common diet myths is something that reads along the lines of "Lose Five Pounds in One Day!" or "The 24-Hour Diet!" You often see these things marketed as tablets, capsules, or liquids. Before you buy into these sorts of scams, or anything where someone is trying to make money off of you, keep in mind not just the information they're offering but also what they're not. In the above sales pitches the goal is clear: weight loss. What's not mentioned is where the weight comes from.

Any time you lose weight in a brief period of hours, it's going to be fluids. Your body can contain several pounds of expendable fluids. Most of these "magic" supplements contain ingredients that are natural or synthetic diuretics, which means they cause you to expel the water in your system. When it's gone, the scale may say you're several pounds lighter but the image in the mirror will look markedly different than if those same pounds had come from fat loss. And, to make matters worse, you'll probably feel one or more side effects of dehydration, which on the simple side can include a headache, fatigue, and dizziness, and on the more complicated side can become a serious health problem. To finish off the bad news, as soon as you drink anything, you're going to put that weight right back on. The moral of the story, as you'll see with the Swimmer's Nutrition Program, is to throw away the scale. We use the mirror, because that's the only thing that matters. The way you look and feel is much more important than any number you have to look down to see.

Another myth is that if you starve yourself, you'll achieve rapid weight loss. This is another situation where you're not getting the whole story. Again you need to ask, Where is the weight coming from? Is it water, fat, or muscle? When you don't eat, your body burns a combination of fat and muscle. Your physical composition largely controls what goes first, but generally it's your hard-earned muscle that is going to be consumed straightaway. Lacking the proper nutrients to feed it, the body goes into a state called catabolism. Literally, your body is eating its own muscle to stay functional. It's very important to remember that not eating is not a good option. You lose muscle as well as much-needed energy.

One important thing to remember about starvation is that the body will always do what it has to in order to stay alive. That goes highly against the thought that not eating will cause a great degree of fat loss. Yes, a certain amount of weight will certainly be lost, but it won't be the kind you're after. The human body knows what it wants, much more than any of us realizes, and it will do everything to protect itself. Many processes in the body severely slow down when starvation is in effect, and that includes the metabolism. There are countless people, and swimmers are no exception to this, who eat very little—often in the range of 500 to 1,000 calories a day—work out for several hours daily, and yet still maintain a high percentage of body fat. If you ask them about it, they're almost always confused as to why this is so. The answer is that because they don't eat, their metabolism is running at a slow pace. That's right, they're overweight because they don't eat enough. It's one of the oddities in life, but it makes a lot of sense.

There are a certain number of calories the body needs to survive on a day-to-day basis. If you're an athlete, that need is greater. So you can see why being an athlete and consuming less than the daily nutritional requirements of a toddler can entirely disrupt the natural course of the body. What happens is that anytime someone on such a deficit eats, the body is so used to being starved that it stores the little food it does get as fat. Fat is like the shield of the body. It has to have it. When there's a consistent source of good, sufficient calories coursing through the system, the body will let it go because it's comfortable "knowing" that more are coming and it will be okay. When that steady source is removed, though, the system goes on the ultimate defensive. Muscle the body can spare a great deal of; fat it won't. We'll get even further into this in the Baseline Diet section when we discuss why eating three meals a day just doesn't cut it.

Alongside the celebrity liquid diets, which really just cause a lot of gastrointestinal discomfort and frequent trips to the bathroom, you'll see "fat loss" pills advertised everywhere from television to magazines to the sides of city buses. While these aren't as bad as some other things that promise results in less than a day, they are also too often littered with lies. Here's what you need to know about weight-loss pills, also known as "thermogenics" or "weight-loss aids."

The human body is a very resilient machine when you think of all the processes it has to handle and the manner in which it works. The metabolism is like a furnace. The food put into the body is what the fire has to burn. As with any open flame, there's only so much that can be burned at once. And, if you really oversaturate it, you can nearly extinguish the flame.

There are several complicated methods to determine your exact metabolism, which you can find through tests available at many health clinics and gyms. While these aren't necessary, some people would like to find out. An easier way to find a general starting point will be explained in the Baseline Diet section later as we start creating your personal program. Just know at this point that your body tries to adapt to the amount of calories provided by increasing or decreasing the metabolism, depending on what you eat.

If, for example, you eat 2,500 calories a day, your body will try to adjust to that standard. Naturally, the body can't increase its metabolism indefinitely, which is where we encounter the problem of putting on body fat. The metabolism, though, is not affected just by your dietary habits, it's also affected by the makeup of what you eat, as well as any stimulants you consume. Caffeine is a good example.

It isn't to be said that the use of these stimulants is ineffective. In fact, ephedra is quite likely the most effective fat-loss aid known to man and was used responsibly and effectively for hundreds, if not thousands, of years before it was abused and subsequently regulated. For most people, though, the use of these stimulants provides only a temporary benefit because they are unaware of how to properly adjust when they are no longer taking them in. The reason is that the body adjusts its metabolism when it realizes there is a caloric deficit (which is necessary when the goal is fat loss). A calorie deficit is defined as burning more calories than you consume. When stimulants are taken in to assist, though, the body further adjusts and can potentially slow its natural rate. For that reason, we're avoiding them and not suggesting they be used in conjunction with the Swimmer's Nutrition Program. Your goals can all be achieved without them.

From here on you're going to see the terms "fat loss" and "weight loss," but realize that they are not the same thing. Our goal is "fat loss" because, remember, we threw out the scale and don't care much about weight. "Weight loss" will literally refer to a change in numbers on a scale and be used only sparsely.

## NUTRITIONAL REQUIREMENTS

We now understand that fat loss and weight loss are very different things. We know our goal is fat loss. Now we need to understand how to achieve that, because weight loss can occur through several avenues, one of which requires the sacrifice of muscle, which is most definitely a negative outcome. Our ultimate goal is not just to induce fat loss but ultimately to readjust our entire body composition. That means we're going to burn the fat and increase the muscle.

Different types of foods provide different benefits and thus are partner to different types of results. One example is that when you're adjusting your diet for weight loss, you'll reduce your carbohydrates slightly while elevating your protein intake slightly. And you'll also find that one of the main attributes of the Swimmer's Nutrition Program is nutrient timing. That is to say, what's important isn't always what you eat but when you eat it. Many people are very excited when they hear that simple sugar does indeed have a place in a proper diet that is combined with exercise.

Carbohydrates have been made out to be Public Enemy No. 1 thanks to the proliferation of certain fad diets. Unfortunately, this evil branding has gone way too far. There are exceptions to every rule, and carbohydrates certainly have their share, but athletes, especially swimmers, need carbohydrates for energy. Again, think of the body as a machine and carbohydrates as one type of fuel. Like grades of gasoline, though, some foods—including carbs—are more "premium" than others.

Protein is a vital component of the muscles of the body but, again unlike in other diets, should not be preached as the only necessity in nutrition. You do need protein, and athletes tend to need more than most people, but that's often because athletes simply need more food in general than other people. For the individual with fat loss in mind, protein helps spare the muscle while burning the fat. We realize that this may seem like a lot of information to take in at once, but the idea is to educate you in simple terms about how the body works. The more you understand your body, the easier it will be for you to make this program work for you and help you achieve your goals faster. As we go on we will be explaining not just what should be done but also why. Hopefully, this will provide not only better results but an even greater sense of satisfaction.

## THE BASELINE DIET—WHERE YOUR BODY IS NOW

Assuming you know your goal (if you don't, keep reading and we'll help you figure it out), the first step in achieving your goal is finding out where you stand nutritionally.

The body adjusts its metabolic rate depending on a person's regular eating habits and physical activity. There's a very simple way to figure out where you stand, without any fancy technology.

For three days, you're going to write down everything you eat. Here's an early warning: Be sure you're doing this when your diet won't be altered from the norm for any reason. If you're traveling, it's not a good idea to start this if it's going to run through that disrupted schedule. Also, you need to make sure you don't change your habits just because you're writing them down. The number one reason body composition changes are delayed is because people "fib" on their baseline diets. Be honest with yourself, because that's the way you're going to get results.

For three days calculate the following:

Food (what you ate) | How Much | Calories (total) | Time of Day

## Guide

Food (what you ate): This is merely what you ate. If you ate pizza, write it down and be sure to include any toppings you may have had.

How Much: A common mistake is writing down the serving suggestion size and not the actual amount you ate. It's generally because people look at the box and see that, for example, a serving of Cheerios is 1 cup and contains 110 calories. Remember, very few people actually eat single servings of things that come out of multiserving packages.

Calories (total): Make sure when you're writing this down that you write the total number of calories and not just the per-serving amount. If you're eating 2 cups of our Cheerios example, then your total is about 220 calories because you ate twice a standard serving. If you're eating something that isn't out of a package, you can often find the number of calories by doing a quick search on the Internet (www.calorie-count.com) or, if you're eating pizza as mentioned before, you can check the website of the company you ordered from and they will have it there.

Time of Day: Pretty self-explanatory; just make a note of what time you ate whatever it was you ate.

Here's a brief example of part of a day:

| Food | How Much | Calories (Total) | Time |
|---|---|---|---|
| Berry yogurt | 8 oz. | 120 | 7 a.m. |
| Eggs | 5 whole | 350 | 8 a.m. |
| Snickers | 1 bar | 280 | 10 a.m. |
| Turkey sandwich | White bread, turkey, cheese, mustard | 310 | 11 a.m. |

After you calculate your three days' worth of calories, you will divide by three. For example, if you consumed 3,000 calories on Day 1, 3,500 on Day 2, and 4,000 on Day 3, your baseline diet is 3,500 calories.

After you've determined your average intake, divide by five. Our goal is to eat at least five times each day at an equal number of calories. In our example, 3,500 is broken down to five meals of 700 calories each.

The reason you will divide meals is that you want to provide your body with a constant source of nutrients. If you eat only two or three times each day, the body becomes used to hoarding what it needs to survive. It's a resiliency it has developed over time to protect itself, but it can be detrimental when it comes to positively altering body composition.

## FAT LOSS

If you're looking to lose fat, you're going to slowly scale back the number of calories you're taking in. This process takes place on a triweekly basis and can provide noticeable, healthy fat loss over a fairly short period of time.

You have to remember that this isn't a miracle diet. There's nothing special about this; it's just working with your body as nature intended. Taking it slow is best, and it's the best way to keep the fat away permanently.

Adjustments are easy, and someone with the baseline of our example could go as follows:

| | |
|---|---|
| Week 1 | 3,500 calories a day |
| Week 4 | 3,250 calories a day |
| Week 7 | 3,000 calories a day |
| Week 10 | 2,750 calories a day |
| Week 13 | 2,500 calories a day |

As you see, everything is done gradually. By doing so, the body can adapt and, most important, can shed practically all body fat while retaining muscle mass. If you do too much too soon, the body will let go of mass, as it's the most dispensable.

Calories are cut by 250 each period so that the body can adapt. Cut calories until you reach the number that puts you at the healthy weight you're after and satisfies your energy requirements. If your fat loss halts early, you can move to the next step. If you're losing more than two pounds each week, you should add some calories to slow things down a bit. Stay mindful that all of your new swimming will burn a lot of calories, so adjust accordingly.

While going through this course, be sure that you're eating enough carbohydrates and fats to maintain a healthy energy level, but be sure you consume protein in higher proportions to help protein synthesis in the body.

## WEIGHT GAIN

Some people have a metabolism to be envious of. No matter what they eat, they just can't put on quality weight. Other people who burn off calories quickly have the problem that when they do eat enough to gain weight, it's fat weight and not muscle.

To rectify this situation, you merely go the reverse of the fat-loss

### Olympian Tip Taming a Sweet Tooth

***Gabe Woodward—***
***bronze medalist, 2004 Athens Olympics***

I have a terrible sweet tooth! Always have and still do. I am trying to tame it, though. Nutritionally, the best way to keep the body healthy is to eat lots of fruits and vegetables. My wife got me a juicer, so I try to juice a few mornings each week. When I'm in heavy training, I try to juice every morning. Whole foods are the best way to go. God made food the best way—the fresher, the better. The more refining and cooking we do to food, the worse we make it for us.

schedule. Instead of cutting caloric intake, you increase it slowly from your baseline. Over time, you will find the right number that will positively influence your body composition. Again, by doing things slowly in combination with a proper workout program, you will add muscle instead of unsightly fat.

For example, we know that eating a candy bar isn't going to help pack on pounds of lean muscle. The nutrient profile of most "junk food" is hardly populated with things our body needs to grow lean tissue. So even if you're one of those people who can't seem to put on any weight no matter what you eat, when you find the right calorie count, eventually you will. But if it's junk food, the calories—the sugars and fats and the like—are going to get stored around the midsection, thighs, etc. . . . But if you add in quality proteins, fats, and carbohydrates from things such as lean meats and slow-burning carbohydrates and healthy fats, your body will put it right to use for quality muscle building.

To offer an example, if your body is burning 2,800 calories a day and you're eating 2,200 or so regularly, slowly start adding in more good food. Doing so slowly will allow your stomach to adjust to taking in more food, and the quality of the substances will help energize you and help craft the physique you're looking for.

## THE RIGHT FOODS

Naturally, calories aren't the only thing you have to watch out for. Calculating your intake is important, but the composition of that intake is vital, too.

You will shortly see a list of quality foods that your body will love you for. Use these as the basis for your nutritional program. We're constantly asked if treats are allowed on occasion; the answer, of course, is yes. Eating ice cream or pizza every once in a while won't—as shocked as some may be to hear this—hurt you. But chances are that after you adapt to a new eating style, you'll crave these foods less and less. Whether you treat yourself or not, keep in mind all the while what it is you're eating and what your goals are.

You want to establish a balanced ratio of protein, carbohydrates, and fats. If you're looking to lose fat, a ratio of 50/30/20 (50% of calories from protein, 30% from carbohydrates, 20% from fats) is good for many while others prefer a 40/30/30 diet. You'll be able to find out what works best for you fairly shortly. You'll notice that carbohydrates don't dominate fat-burning programs, neither here nor in other "mainstream" diets. Carbohydrates aren't evil, but they can bulk up your waistline if you're not careful because of their makeup. If you're very sensitive to the effects of carbohydrates, that is to say your body likes to hold on to fat stores when you're taking in large amounts of them, cut them back a bit.

If you find that your energy is constantly running low, subtract 5–10% protein and replace it with carbohydrates. You can adjust again at a later time as well. Over time you will learn what works best for your body.

## NUTRIENTS AND THEIR SOURCES

Probably the most commonly asked question when we're working with teams, or even individual athletes, on the topic of nutrition is

"What do you eat before a race?" Or "What do you eat the morning of a competition?" Often there are half a dozen variants of this same question at any presentation.

Rather than just provide answers as to what some of the best foods before a race or a training session are, we would like to explain why it is you need certain foods. As mentioned earlier in this book, you should always know why you're doing something.

The general principle, as we have said, is timing the nutrients properly. Here's a list of important nutrients, what they are, and sample sources of each.

## Simple Carbohydrates

These are simple, single-molecule sugars. They consists of monosaccharides (such as glucose and fructose) and disaccharides (such as sucrose, maltose, and lactose) and should generally be avoided.

### Sample Simple Carbohydrate Sources

Cakes
Ham
Chocolate
Candy
Honey
Cola
White bread

## Complex Carbohydrates

These are found in starchy foods and fiber sources, and are broken down more slowly than simple carbohydrates to provide longer-lasting energy. Chemically, complex carbohydrates have a more complicated structure than their "simple" counterparts.

### Sample Complex Carbohydrate Sources

| | |
|---|---|
| Grains | Lentils |
| Whole wheat bread | Oatmeal |
| Pasta | Brown rice |
| Vegetables | Bran |
| Peas | Muesli |
| Beans | |

## Protein

Protein is made up of amino acids, which are often called the building blocks of muscle. Protein is the major structural component of all lean tissue in the body and is necessary for the growth of new muscle tissue as well as the repair of current muscle tissue.

### Sample Protein Sources

| | |
|---|---|
| Chicken | Halibut |
| Turkey | Tuna |
| Ground beef | Milk |
| Salmon | |

## Fats

Another of the main classes of foods, fats are multipurpose and come in saturated and unsaturated forms. Saturated fats (most often found in animal products) are linked to increased levels of arteriosclerosis (hardening of the arteries), while unsaturated fats can be used as a source of energy and have many uses in the body.

Fats are needed by the body and carry fat-soluble vitamins as well as supplying the body with essential fatty acids.

### Sample Saturated Fat Sources

| | |
|---|---|
| Coconut oil | Whole milk |
| Palm oil | Cream |
| Butter | Animal meats |
| Cheeses | |

### Sample Unsaturated Fat Sources

| | |
|---|---|
| Nuts | Seeds |
| Olives | Olive oil |
| Fatty fish (e.g., salmon) | |

Now that you have an understanding of the three classes of foods that the body needs and an idea of what they do, it is easier to understand why certain foods are better at certain times of the day and before various activities, and why some foods should be avoided altogether.

## NUTRIENT TIMING

One of the main things we focus on when designing a nutrition program is the timing of the meal. Just about everything you'll take in will be considered a meal, as snacks are generally understood as small, simple "fillers" just to get you by. When you're training and trying to build muscle or burn fat, you'll need different foods at different times to make the progress you're after.

To give you an idea of why nutrient timing is important, think of an activity you're going to set out to do, maybe a big goal after training for a few months, like completing a long open-water swim. If you were to wake up and go right out and swim, what would happen? You'd tire quickly because you hadn't eaten and properly fueled your body for the exercise. As opposed to that, if you had eaten a solid protein source like eggs and a slow-digesting carbohydrate source like brown rice, you would have a long-sustained source of fuel. Enough fuel, in fact, that pretty quickly you'd be passing those who didn't prepare correctly.

With that knowledge, you'll want to apply those exact principles of preparation after a workout and even before bed as well. Each activity may require different foods, but knowing when to take them in makes a great deal of difference when it comes down to how that nutrition manifests itself in the form of benefits: energy, strength, and endurance.

One manner of putting together a proper nutrition program is to cut out foods that aren't necessary for the body. As one would imagine, to do this completely is nearly impossible, but the good news is that you don't absolutely have to avoid things like saturated fat. A healthy choice is to avoid it when possible, but the small amounts in foods like 1% milk won't do any significant cumulative harm when taken in moderation.

So we now know the body needs carbohydrates, protein, and fats. Since carbohydrates and fats are sources of energy, used by the body when put under different stresses, while protein is responsible mainly for the repair and construction of new lean tissue, we have a general understanding of how to put together a full day of meals based on what different foods do.

Before getting too specific regarding dietary needs, it should be understood that nutrition, and the human body, are complicated things. There's so much information surrounding vitamins, micronutrients, fats, and so on that it would be impossible to include it all in one book. In fact, there are things about food that scientists admit we probably don't even know about. Our goal here is not necessarily to be the study material for a 400-level nutrition class, but instead to teach you how to adapt your eating habits for your own optimal health and performance.

There are several factors that influence the various foods you should eat at different points in the day, such as length of time between meals, type of activity, composition of prior meals, and individual metabolism.

## Pre-workout

If you're getting ready for a workout, you have to take into account what you're going to be doing. The average workout, regardless of sport, usually works all types of muscle fibers, taxes your body's glycogen stores, calls upon fat for fuel, and pushes you hard for long periods of time. To give your body the best chance of (figuratively) surviving these tests of fortitude, you have to give it the right fuel. You wouldn't expect to see the world's best race car drivers putting cheap and inadequate fuel into the engines of their high-priced, top-of-the-line vehicles, so don't do it to yourself.

Carbohydrates (glucose) are stored as glycogen in the body. During exercise, these stores are called upon at higher intensity levels. Because fats are broken down and put to use slowly, they are usually burned during lower-intensity exercise. Because workouts consist of both low- and high-intensity sets, you need both in your pre-workout meal, with fats being consumed in lesser quantities. Protein, a source of amino acids and the major component of muscle, should also be consumed to keep up your strength and round out a well-balanced meal that will prepare your body for the stress that will ensue.

A quality breakfast would include things like whole grains, whole wheat bread, and oatmeal (but not the instant kind) as sources of carbohydrates.

Peanut butter is an example of a tasty source of unsaturated fat, assuming you choose an organic brand.

Organic foods in general are good options, but you have to remember that in most countries the rules aren't very clear on what can and can't be considered organic. Often, people pay three or even four times the amount of a similar product simply because it says "organic" and it's really of no better quality than the alternative. But as a practice, remember that the more food is altered—frozen, cooked, fried, processed—the more nutrients are taken away. As such, we encourage you to get foods as fresh as possible and cook them as soon as possible.

When thinking of your protein needs, yogurt and fat-free or low-fat milk are choices of dairy products that also provide fat. Eggs are not only a good source of protein but also the most obvious breakfast food.

Something worth considering is your approach to breakfast. What do you consider breakfast food? Many bodybuilders eat chicken, steak, or fish every morning. They eat oatmeal at what most people consider "dinnertime." Oatmeal is a food that most people enjoy, but simply at a later time of the day. Don't forget that the nutritional value of a food doesn't change, so if you enjoy it and don't mind having it within your first meal or two of the day, you should give it a try.

### During Workout

Generally, in the realm of exercise nutrition, people think of only "pre" and "post" exercise nutrition. By doing so they're missing out on a very valuable opportunity to replenish the body and increase peak performance. Science has told us that glycogen stores are about depleted when exercise exceeds 45 to 60 minutes, leaving the body with less functional fuel to use. At this point, something like a single carbohydrate gel packet or sixteen to thirty-two ounces of a carbohydrate drink is of great benefit to the training athlete. Another commonly marketed option is bars. Gatorade and PowerBar both make several of these products, but we generally recommend against them during and immediately after exercise because they take much longer to break down and become useful. Thus we consider the other options superior choices for consumption during strenuous activity.

Of the gels and drinks you can find or make on your own, it generally comes down to a personal choice. Which do you prefer? Both are quickly broken down, and both—if made of quality ingredients—will help you fight off fatigue during long sessions of training. Even Gummi Bears can come through in a pinch.

For some people, drinks with high sugar content can be upsetting to their stomach. If this happens to you, don't worry—it isn't uncommon and may very well make the decision—gel or drink—easier to reach.

Oddly enough, some coaches still hate to see their athletes taking in these types of carbohydrate supplements. Some say that they're nothing more than marketing, while others take more of an "old-school" approach and assume that if they didn't need them, no one does. Luckily, science has disproved the initial argument, and a slew of world records in all sports over the past decade may push away the latter. One study conducted back in 1983 by the American Physiological Society, well before the vast majority of marketed supplements hit the shelves, found that carbohydrate supplementation during exercise greatly increased the amount of time it took athletes to reach a level of fatigue that altered their performance. Countless studies since have proven those same results.

### Post-workout

By the time a workout is over, whether it was an hour of lifting weights, a two-hour swim, or running long distances preparing for a triathlon or marathon, the body has used up its glycogen stores and many muscle fibers have been broken down and are in need of repair. Fats, being the most abundant source of fuel in the body and more slowly broken down, are of less importance at this stage.

Immediately after a workout, exercising athletes should be on a mission to repair the damage done. It's the best thing one can do to prepare himself or herself to come back better next time. You want fast-acting sources of carbohydrates, and you want amino acids that can be put to work right away to repair lean tissue.

Many athletes have a favorite brand of protein powder that they like to take after exercise. This is a great start; a whey protein powder is a fast-acting, easily and quickly digested nutrient source that will go a good way toward repairing your muscles. Unfortunately, it isn't enough. It's like getting dressed and forgetting to put your shoes on: you're missing something. Most protein shakes don't have much sugar, which is generally a good thing at other points of the day. After intense training, though, you want something to blunt any catabolism—muscle breakdown—taking place in the body.

There are some good options out there pertaining to products that include carbohydrates and protein together, but these are often highly touted as some miracle supplement (which they aren't) and thus are quite costly. If you want to go the shake route, which is used with great results by countless elite athletes, a simple solution is to buy your favorite brand of plain whey protein powder and add dextrose sugar, which is the food industry name for the biologically active form of glucose, a monosaccharide.

Regular table sugar is a disaccharide and its technical name is sucrose. Because of the structural difference, plain cane sugar has to be broken down into glucose before use. As such, it makes more sense, to aid in the quickest recovery, to ingest the simplest form of sugar with your post-workout shake. You can find this in some food stores, but also online at a variety of retailers.

Many people dislike the taste of protein powders, calling them "chalky" or simply not caring for the artificial flavors many possess. For these people, another beneficial drink to take in (remember, liquids are easier to digest than whole foods and thus superior in this situation) is a yogurt drink. Yoplait makes Nouriche and Dannon has created Frusion. Generally these products contain a 4:1 ratio of carbohydrates to protein, which is called the "optimum blend" by many nutrition experts.

So at this point we're going to assume you have your favorite food picked out to have in your bag, or at least somewhere readily available, as soon as you hop out of the pool. Don't be afraid to mix it up every once in a while; even if you find something you like, it's a good idea to go with something else you like for a couple days here and there. That way, you don't get bored with it. There isn't much worse in the nutrition realm than finding some delicious, nutritious food that you soon begin to pass on because you tire of it. Ask any competitive bodybuilder how he feels about chicken and broccoli, and you'll quickly understand!

While the intake of nutrients immediately after you finish your exercise session is fairly important, true post-workout nutrition is only beginning at this stage. Your muscles don't grow (or repair) while they're under stress—as when working out—so you have to give them what they need when they do have the opportunity to regenerate. That time is between workouts. Equally important after that initial liquid intake of nutrients is a whole-food meal rich in complex carbohydrates and solid proteins. At this point, adding a little fat into your meal isn't a real issue, but fats do slow the digestive process and for that reason we generally suggest keeping them to a minimum right after working out and in the first full meal afterward.

As mentioned in the breakfast section, if it's something you enjoy, there's really no food that can be eaten only at a certain time of day. That said, eggs are again a great choice here, as are brown rice, potatoes, fish, and chicken. Take this meal sixty to ninety minutes after you finish your liquid meal.

## Before Bed

The final meal of the day is often the most neglected in many respects: it's the one you take right before going to bed. When should it be eaten? What should it consist of? When these are answered, the next question is "Why?"

People tend to look at sleep as a peaceful time, a time of "nothing," because aside from their dreams, they don't consider it a stage where much happens. That opinion is actually about as far from the truth as one could get. Sure, you dream, but the body undergoes more repair and growth during sleep than it ever could while awake.

Many people have heard of human growth hormone. It usually gets a bad rap—maybe you just saw on television another athlete busted for cheating with it—or it's marketed as some wonder drug for those wanting to fight aging. In any case, a certain amount of this hormone occurs naturally in the body and can provide a host of benefits when allowed to do so.

Human growth hormone in the body is secreted by the pituitary gland. Its principal functions are to stimulate not only growth, as the name suggests, but cell repair. The major release of this hormone in the body takes place after you fall asleep. During sleep, the body also tries to repair the muscles, rest the mind, and revitalize after a hard day. Obviously, the more sleep (to an extent) you get, the better you feel. But still, even after a continuous eight hours of sleep, many people—especially athletes—wake up feeling weak and tired. Generally, this is because their bodies have been breaking down during the night instead of building up. This happens because proper nutrients haven't been fed to the body for several hours.

Because you don't eat during sleep, your body can use only what it has on hand. Effectively, your repair during sleep is about as productive as your last meal. Was it rich in nutrients, or was it something high in insulin-spiking sugar like ice cream?

As you've seen, proper nutrition involves a vast change from the traditional "three square meals" model. If you eat breakfast upon waking, lunch at noon, and dinner after work, you're really at a disadvantage because on top of those eight hours of sleep, you didn't eat in the three or four hours you were last awake.

Truth be told, there's very little you can do this side of intravenous injection—which is obviously not an option—to provide your body with amino acids throughout the course of an entire night's rest. What you can do, though, is give your body the best possible source of vitamins and minerals prior to bed that, if taken in the proper forms, can slowly break down and trickle into your system while you rest.

Eating before bed has been known to cause problems for some people in the form of stomach discomfort. Sometimes this is because the timing is new to their body, and it will go away after a couple of days' practice. Others merely can't handle the influx of food before lying flat on their backs for hours at a time. In general, though, people are receptive to this new meal. If you're not, practice with different foods until you find one that works for you, because there's bound to be something available.

We talked earlier about nutrient timing when it had to do with workouts. As you see, there's no difference before sleep. You need the right nutrients at the right time.

Protein supports muscle growth, carbohydrates promote active energy, and fats are a source of fuel and vitamins. At this stage, because we aren't preparing the body for stress, the two most important food classes are going to be protein and fats. Fats, again, have the added benefit of slowing digestion, which further slows the breakdown of food, and offers the advantage of providing your body nutrients for a longer period of time.

An excellent example choice for a bedtime meal is cottage cheese eaten about 15 minutes before bed because it's high in protein that is derived from milk and is therefore slowly released. Other options include caseinate protein powders and skim milk.

### Middle of the Night

This following tip is really only for the most serious of trainers, as it's certainly not mandatory, but it's a feasible step of the program that you can add if you want. We do it ourselves, but whether or not you do is completely an individual choice.

Taking a casein protein before bed is about as good as you can do for yourself before depriving yourself of food for, hopefully, eight to nine hours of sleep. Eventually, though, that slow trickle of amino acids runs out and you're running on empty for a couple of hours. However, if your sleep is interrupted for some reason and you wake up in the middle of the night, whether because the dog is barking or you just have to use the bathroom, you can grab a quick, small snack to give your body some more nutrients.

At the point you would do this, even a whey protein is feasible. Some people drink a quick protein shake, others eat a hard-boiled egg or two, others consume a few ounces of cold skim milk or cottage cheese. The difference is really quite noticeable when you wake up to start your day: you're not starving because your body was given more nutrition to help it recover and build muscle.

A couple of things to look out for are that if you're trying to lose weight, make sure you count these calories. Just because you may be a bit sleepy when you eat them doesn't mean they don't count. Second, don't eat anything in the middle of the night that will keep you from returning to sleep. Something very small is all you need, because the benefit of doing this won't outweigh a lost hour of sleep if you have to wait for your stomach to settle before getting back into bed.

Last, don't set your alarm for this. Uninterrupted sleep is by far the best nightly choice; this tip is just an option to make the best of a bad situation.

## WHAT'S NOT NUTRITION

A lot of people are preached a practice of moderation. They're often told that things like sweets are okay if they're consumed only in small servings, and not too often. Generally, this is an acceptable practice. After all, eating something that tastes exceptionally good is satisfying on a lot of levels.

Despite the innocence of an occasional treat, there are still some things you should stay away from. And for the time being, while these ingredients may be in your favorite cheat foods, they're really worth avoiding.

### Hydrogenated Oils

Hydrogenated oils are among the worst food additives you can consume. In fact, the debate against them reached a fever pitch in 2006, when some states were considering banning their use entirely. Luckily, many fast-food chains have already eliminated their use.

These oils, also listed as "partially hydrogenated" oils, are created through a process of adding hydrogen to the base. They assist in keeping foods fresher, longer, and more stable. If you've ever wondered why you have to stir most natural peanut butters, it is because they don't contain this ingredient.

Hydrogenated oils create dangerous "trans fat," which is a term you've probably heard of thanks to increasing media coverage. This by-product fat has been shown to have a negative effect on lipid profiles and increases the risk of coronary heart disease.

### Simple Sugars

Simple sugars have been discussed as having a value when consumed post-workout, to prevent the possibility of catabolism in the muscles. That said, they're otherwise bad for your health due to the resulting insulin spike, which promotes fat storage and negative blood sugar levels. Fibrous carbohydrates such as those found in vegetables generally have a fiber content that slows their digestion and increases the likelihood that they will be burned as fuel. Simple sugars, like fructose, should as a rule be avoided whenever possible.

### Artificial Sweeteners

Artificial sweeteners, such as aspartame and sucralose, have been debated as to how safe they really are. Some studies show an increased risk of Alzheimer's disease with the intake of aspartame, for example, while others deny this risk. In any case, artificial sweeteners, like artificial foods, are things our bodies weren't designed to metabolize. When possible, use less of the real stuff instead.

Technology and the desire to have everything faster have largely prevented us all from eating the way God intended for us. Even given that truth, technology has also made otherwise hard-to-get nutrients readily available to us. There's certainly a give-and-take, and there's still plenty we can do to improve our health. Eating as best we can with the foods available to us is a start; avoiding the foods we know to be most harmful to us is another step in the right direction. For most people, just changing the way they eat, even before getting involved with an exercise program, will create dramatic changes in their physiques. They'll look better, but most important, they will feel better, which will allow a greater appreciation of life and all of the wonderful things it has to offer!

## SUPPLEMENTS THAT WORK

With a proper diet, the average active individual does not necessarily need any dietary supplementation. That said, there are a few simple, healthful things that can be added to your nutritional program to enhance your well-being.

Many times people forget the meaning behind the word "supplement." Please keep in mind that the products mentioned below will be of little good if not accompanied by an adequate intake of quality foods.

### $CoQ_{10}$

Coenzyme Q-10, more commonly called $CoQ_{10}$, is a powerful antioxidant that helps eliminate free radicals from the body. This supplement has also been shown to help improve cardiovascular function and reduce blood pressure, and it plays a key role in energy production in the body as well.

## EPA/DHA (Docosahexaenoic Acid and Eicosapentaenoic Acid)

This supplement and its long-form name is a fancy way to say fish oil, essential omega-3 fatty acids. The benefits of this supplement are numerous, and they include improved brain function, improved cardiovascular function, enhanced lipid profile, and improved body composition as the fatty acids promote the shedding of body fat stores.

As more of the world's waterways become polluted, there are reports coming to light that show high levels of mercury in the supply of fish humans consume. While the amount of fish that most people eat isn't enough to worry about, by supplementing your diet with pill-form fish oil you're reducing one worry while taking advantage of all the available benefits.

## Vitamin C

There is some research to suggest that active individuals may have low levels of vitamin C in their bodies. The *International Journal of Sport Nutrition and Exercise Metabolism* published a study in 2006 showing that vitamin C supplementation can increase fat oxidation during submaximal aerobic exercise, as well as help "reduce muscle soreness, damage, function and oxidative stress due to eccentric exercise."

As a suggestion, taking 500 mg each day of this vitamin could be beneficial to your health and exercise performance.

## Amino Acids

The *International Journal of Sport Nutrition and Exercise Metabolism* published another study, this one in December 2006, on the use of amino acids and their effect on muscle soreness. They found that when consumed thirty minutes prior to and immediately after exercise, muscle soreness was considerably lower than in the placebo group of their test. One serving before and after exercise is recommended.

## Creatine

For years there has been a great deal of misinformation surrounding this product, which is actually naturally occurring in the body. It is not a steroid—it is an amino acid—and it has never been proven dangerous to otherwise healthy adults. In fact, creatine has been proven safe throughout thousands of studies and has been proven to promote increases in lean body mass, positive body composition, muscular strength and even brain function—2 to 5 grams a day is sufficient.

13

# Recipes

The recipes we've included here—which we enjoy while training—are reminders that you don't have to go out to eat tasty meals. They're easy and delicious and with the right timing will help prepare you for physical activity or recovery. This will also show you that there can be much variety while sticking to some basic building blocks, like chicken and turkey.

Don't be surprised that this menu includes carbohydrates. Remember, this book is an entire program—exercise, stretching, and nutrition—and the body needs carbohydrates for fuel. Don't be afraid of them. While cutting carbs may be the latest trend, it isn't what we're after. Swimmers burn up carbohydrates by the figurative truckload, so you'll need to replenish them in order to stay feeling energized and healthy.

Keep in mind that all information pertaining to these recipes is approximate.

# BREAKFAST

**Egg and Cheese Breakfast Sandwich**

1 whole wheat English muffin

2 large eggs

1 slice fat-free American cheese

Toast English muffin and scramble 1 whole egg and 1 egg white. Just before eggs are done, center them in pan, place cheese on top, and cover until cheese begins to melt. Place on muffin.

1 SERVING

EACH SERVING: 240 CALORIES, 30 G CARBOHYDRATES, 19 G PROTEIN

**Breakfast Yogurt**

1 cup fat-free vanilla yogurt

½ cup granola

1 cup mixed berries

Combine ingredients. Can also be a post-workout meal. Here's a tip: Save your 8 oz. yogurt cups that come in store-bought, pre-made blends, and afterward buy bulk yogurt and refill the cups with your own creations.

1 SERVING

EACH SERVING: 300 CALORIES, 55 G CARBOHYDRATES, 12 G PROTEIN

**Grilled Chicken Salad**

1 boneless, skinless chicken breast

2–4 cups salad mix

2 ounces feta cheese

2 tablespoons fat-free dressing

Salt and pepper to taste

Grill chicken until cooked through and cut into thin strips or small squares. Top salad mix with chicken. Sprinkle cheese on top and add dressing.

EACH SERVING: 350 CALORIES, 16 TO 18 G CARBOHYDRATES, 35 G PROTEIN

## LUNCH/DINNER

**Tuna Salad**

1 can tuna in water

1 tablespoon fat-free mayonnaise

2 tablespoons relish

3–5 whole wheat crackers

Drain tuna and place in bowl. Mix in mayo and relish (relish can be substituted with chopped-up pickles). Crumble and mix in crackers.

1 SERVING

EACH SERVING: 200 CALORIES, 8 G CARBOHYDRATES, 30 G PROTEIN

### Grilled Chicken Salad with Asparagus

1 boneless, skinless chicken breast
4 cups lettuce, washed
1 cup cherry tomatoes
¾ pound asparagus spears
¼ cup salad dressing, any kind

Grill chicken until cooked through and cut into thin strips or small squares. Top lettuce with chicken, tomatoes, and asparagus. Add dressing.

EACH SERVING: 310 CALORIES, 10 G CARBOHYDRATES, 35 G PROTEIN

### Grilled Turkey Dijon Salad

1 pound turkey breast tenderloins
1 dozen cherry tomatoes, halved
1 dozen mushrooms, halved
1 small red onion, peeled and sliced into rings
1 red pepper, cut into thin strips
½ cup Dijon mustard
4 cups salad mix
Ground black pepper to taste

Grill turkey until cooked through and cut into 1½ x ¼-inch strips. Combine in large bowl with tomatoes, mushrooms, onion, and pepper. Lightly toss mixture while adding Dijon mustard. Top salad mix with turkey.

4 SERVINGS

EACH SERVING: 290 CALORIES, 10 G CARBOHYDRATES, 30 G PROTEIN

### Lemon Baked Chicken

2 to 3 tablespoons olive oil
3 to 4 tablespoons fresh lemon juice
1 garlic clove, crushed
1½ teaspoons ground black pepper
2 to 3 boneless, skinless chicken breasts

Preheat oven to 350°F. Combine olive oil, lemon juice, garlic, and pepper in a small bowl. Place chicken in baking dish, and pour mixture over to coat. Cover and bake 30 to 35 minutes or until chicken is cooked thoroughly (varies with amount cooked).

2 TO 3 SERVINGS

EACH SERVING: 200 CALORIES, 1 G CARBOHYDRATE, 35 G PROTEIN

### Balsamic Chicken

2 tablespoons olive oil
2 to 3 boneless, skinless chicken breasts
1 green or red pepper, cut into thin strips
1 white onion, sliced
2 garlic gloves, crushed
Balsamic vinegar to taste
Salt and ground black pepper to taste

Place chicken in baking pan. Pour olive oil over chicken. Add pepper, onion, and garlic, and balsamic vinegar. Mix well. Marinate, refrigerated, 30 to 90 minutes. Bake at 375°F until chicken is cooked thoroughly, 30 to 40 minutes.

2 TO 3 SERVINGS

EACH SERVING: 175 CALORIES, 3 G CARBOHYDRATES, 35 G PROTEIN

## Chicken Dijon

¼ cup extra virgin olive oil
1 tablespoon soy sauce
2 garlic cloves, crushed
1 tablespoon minced ginger
1 tablespoon Dijon mustard
6 skinless, boneless chicken breasts
Salt and ground black pepper to taste

Combine olive oil, soy sauce, garlic, ginger, and mustard. Spread or brush mixture over both sides of the chicken. Allow chicken to sit in refrigerator for at least 1 hour. Over medium heat, grill chicken until cooked through. Turn over halfway through cooking.

6 SERVINGS

EACH SERVING: 275 CALORIES, 1 G CARBOHYDRATE, 35 G PROTEIN

## Simple Shrimp

2 tablespoons extra virgin olive oil
6 ounces shrimp, deveined
2 tablespoons paprika

Pour olive oil into pan and add rinsed/cleaned shrimp. Cook on stove over medium heat until done. When shrimp are half cooked, stir in paprika.

1 SERVING

EACH SERVING: 200 CALORIES, 8 G CARBOHYDRATES, 34 G PROTEIN

### Healthy Nachos

2 whole wheat tortillas
8 ounces 99% fat-free ground turkey
2 tablespoons fat-free sour cream
2 tablespoons tomato salsa
Shredded lettuce
Tomato, diced
2 ounces fat-free cheddar cheese, shredded

Cut tortillas into triangles and place on baking sheet (brush with olive oil if desired). Bake until crisp. Cook turkey in pan until done. Place on tortillas on plate. Add sour cream, salsa, lettuce, tomato, and cheese.

SERVINGS

EACH SERVING: 500 CALORIES, 32 G CARBOHYDRATES, 74 G PROTEIN

### Eggs and Beans

7 eggs
½ can black beans
½ cup salsa

Mix 2 whole eggs with 5 egg whites and cook until soft curds are formed. Pour warmed black beans over eggs and stir in salsa. Scoop up on whole wheat tortilla chips if desired.

1 SERVING

EACH SERVING: 390 CALORIES, 30 G CARBOHYDRATES, 36 G PROTEIN

## Turkey Tenderloins

2½ pounds turkey breast tenderloins
½ cup white wine
1 teaspoon garlic, crushed
½ teaspoon thyme leaves, crushed
½ teaspoon salt
½ teaspoon ground black pepper
¼ tablespoon Tabasco sauce
2 cups sliced onion
½ teaspoon sugar

Combine ingredients in Ziploc bag, leaving a cushion of air inside. Toss around to coat and allow to sit in refrigerator at least 4 hours. When ready, remove turkey from bag and place in coated baking dish. Pour marinade over turkey and roast at 325°F until turkey is cooked thoroughly, about 30 minutes.

8 SERVINGS

EACH SERVING: 175 CALORIES, 3 G CARBOHYDRATES, 30 G PROTEIN

## Turkey Parmigiana

2 egg whites
1 tablespoon water
½ cup seasoned bread crumbs
2 tablespoons grated Parmesan cheese
1 cup Italian tomato sauce
1 cup part-skim mozzarella cheese, shredded
1 pound turkey breast cutlets, pounded to even thickness

Preheat oven to 400°F. Mix egg whites with water and beat to combine. In separate bowl, mix bread crumbs and cheese. Place turkey in egg/water mix, then into bread crumb/cheese mix. Place on baking pan and bake for 5 minutes. Pour tomato sauce evenly over turkey and sprinkle cheese on top. Bake an additional 5 minutes or until turkey is cooked thoroughly and cheese is melted.

4 SERVINGS

EACH SERVING: 300 CALORIES, 15 G CARBOHYDRATES, 35 G PROTEIN

## Turkey Breast Diane

Pam spray
1 pound turkey breast cutlets, pounded to even thickness
2 teaspoons lemon pepper seasoning
2 tablespoons lemon juice
1 tablespoon Worcestershire sauce
1 teaspoon Dijon mustard

Spray a sauté pan with Pam spray. Heat pan over medium heat for 30 seconds. Sprinkle both sides of cutlets with lemon pepper and place turkey into heated pan. Add lemon juice. Sauté until cooked thoroughly, about 4 minutes on each side. Combine remaining ingredients in bowl and mix well. Add to pan until heated.

EACH SERVING: 150 CALORIES, 1 G CARBOHYDRATE, 30 G PROTEIN

## Simple Mixes

Cottage cheese and pineapple
Cooked lean ground beef and salsa

## AN EXAMPLE DAY'S DIET PLAN

To give you an actual idea of a full day's meals, here's a sample day of food for Megan. Keep in mind that this diet helps fuel her body specifically, and helps her get the most of three hours of swimming daily along with an hour of weight training. The foods can be of benefit to you as well; just be sure to adjust portions accordingly.

**Meal 1**

1 cup oats

8 ounces yogurt

25g whey protein shake

12 ounces water

**Meal 2**

Chicken salad

12 ounces water

**Meal 3**

1 bagel, light cream cheese

1 whole egg, 3 egg whites

12 ounces water

**Meal 4**

1 cup green grapes

1 can tuna fish with two sliced pickles and mayonnaise

12 ounces water

**Meal 5**

6 ounces flank steak

1 medium potato with sour cream

1 artichoke

12 ounces water

**Meal 6**

4 ounces flank steak

Brown rice

Green beans

Sugar snap peas

12 ounces water

**Meal 7**

8 ounces skim milk

14

# Dryland Training

## GENERAL DRYLAND ADVICE

It never hurts to remind people who are about to undertake a physical fitness routine that it's a good idea to consult with your doctor prior to starting. If you have any ailments or concerns, it is best to address them prior to training. This helps in that you won't have to stop after you get going because of a previously unknown condition, and you'll be sure not to aggravate any problems you might have.

That said, a few general notes should be made about training with weights. First, always warm up properly. Never jump right into high-intensity work if you haven't prepared your body to do so.

Second, breathe. As odd as it sounds, it's really not that uncommon to watch trainers get so caught up in what they're doing that they forget to take in oxygen, and soon they're red in the face and not feeling very well. Breathe normally. Most people are comfortable with expelling air during the contraction phase of an exercise—the part that causes your muscles to work on moving the weight—and breathing in on the negative, where the weight returns to its starting position.

Third, go slow. And we mean that in a couple of different ways. The first being that you should introduce exercises that are new to you only one or two at a time. Don't try to overload your brain, or your body, with too much too soon. Remember, this is a lifelong journey in staying physically fit, so you have the time to get to know these exercises and routines thoroughly and properly. Second, go slow with the actual lifting. Not superslow so that it takes you ten seconds per repetition, but about two to three seconds up and two to three seconds down is good. Don't throw the weights around; move smoothly. You'll get more benefit from working with a twenty-five-pound weight than you will with a fifty-pound weight if you have to use body momentum to move the heavier one. That point leads us into our next tip.

Focus on feeling the muscle work. Whether you're working with weights or doing exercises without them, make a mind-to-muscle connection with your body. Concentrate on what's happening, why it's happening, and focus on the feeling.

Last, don't overdo it. If your body feels thoroughly abused (in a good way) and used up after four sets for a muscle group, then stop right there. You did enough; you did great. Don't listen to anyone who tells you that you *have* to do a certain amount of weight, reps, or sets. This is your body, and only you can tell when you've had enough. The idea is to leave a workout with your body tired and done, in need of recovery, but your mind enthusiastic and ready for your next full effort.

For decades there was a theory that the more you trained, the better you became. If you wanted to be stronger, faster, and more muscular, then training every day was supposedly the key. This ideology had countless people hitting the gym, track, and pool seven days each week and going until they couldn't go anymore. They would wake up tired and sore the next morning and then put in another workout. If they struggled, it was—again, in theory—a sign of weakness. Now we know that just isn't the case.

The term for training too much is now simply called "overtraining." When you reach this point, your body is being put through additional stress before it has recovered from your last training session. By doing so you're putting yourself at a higher risk of injury as well as illness, because when you've been overtraining, your immune system isn't able to operate at its peak.

With that in mind, you need (if you're using this along with our swim training program) to be sure your body is prepared for the rigors of more training. If you're new to the sport of swimming, we highly encourage you to train for several months in the water before adding dryland training. If you're using this guide on its own and you're not a swimmer, just keep in mind that the old mantra of "more is better" doesn't apply here.

## MIMIC THE WATER

If you're looking to improve your swimming, you need to do things on land that will improve the main attributes required for quality swimming.

Think about what you need in the water: flexibility and strength, but most important, muscular endurance. Power lifting isn't going to do much good if your goal is losing body fat and swimming faster. There's a certain amount of heavy training that belongs in any workout program, but by no means should it be the major factor.

We work in phases when it comes to dryland training. First, we look to build strength. Second, we look to build endurance in those now-stronger muscles, which will allow us to actually take advantage of them. If your maximum curl weight is fifteen pounds, curling five pounds for twenty-rep sets will get you only so far. It certainly won't alter your ability to pull water. Our goal is to build your strength up, which will provide plenty of benefits—physically and aesthetically—and then we will move on to making it functional for longer periods. This cycle is repeated, and your fitness level constantly progresses.

Remember, as in any type of training, to progress with dryland (with or without weights) you have to challenge yourself. You can't just keep pressing the weights or doing the exercises that are easy. If you work the exercises that are difficult, they become easy, but you have to keep challenging yourself. That's what makes working out so rewarding, because you can continually watch your progress and measure it both in your training and in the mirror.

## TIMING

If you're training in the pool and with dryland work, we suggest training dryland three days each week with the following split:

| | |
|---|---|
| Day 1 (Monday) | Chest, arms |
| Day 2 (Wednesday) | Legs |
| Day 3 (Saturday) | Back, shoulders |

If there is a time where you cannot get to a pool and you're training only on dry land, we suggest four days a week of training with this split:

| | |
|---|---|
| Day 1 (Monday) | Chest |
| Day 2 (Wednesday) | Back, triceps |
| Day 3 (Friday) | Legs |
| Day 4 (Sunday) | Shoulders, biceps |

The days can be adjusted to your own schedule; just be sure to give yourself at least a day of rest between dryland training days.

If you're the type of person who's always on the go and can't make it to the gym regularly or three to four times each week, we suggest two full-body workouts per week. If that sounds like too little, don't worry, you're still fully capable of getting into the best shape of your life.

## THINGS TO AVOID

Don't put yourself in vulnerable positions. This applies to you foremost if you chose to swim because of its lack of impact. It means a lot of things—you don't want to use weights that are too heavy, you don't want to move into working sets if you haven't warmed up properly, and you don't want to put unnecessary pressure on your joints. All these will defeat the purpose of why you started swimming in the first place.

We are strong opponents of things like stair jumps, weighted jumps, and other techniques that cause a large amount of force to be placed upon the body very suddenly. You always need to be especially careful of your knees because the problems you will encounter after a knee injury can be difficult to rectify. Breaststroke is especially dependent on the knees, and remember, it's the best exercise stroke in the pool, so it wouldn't be good for your pool training if you couldn't do it.

If you enjoy running, we're certainly not telling you not to continue training on the track or street. But if you're into exercises that put you at a greater risk of injury, we would much rather see you get the same training benefits from other, safer exercises.

## EXERCISES

All of the exercises here are safe for swimmers and are part of many elite athletes' programs. You'll notice here that all free-weight exercises are done with dumbbells, which we feel is an important safety issue. While barbells can certainly be a healthy method of weight training, we prefer individual free weights, as they offer less restriction and a fuller range of motion. Ultimately this places less stress on joints, which is extremely important, and it also allows any flaws in strength symmetry to be corrected.

Before getting into your working sets—a set is a completion of a predetermined number of repetitions on any of these exercises, be sure to do a warm-up set with much lighter weights than you'll use in your main sets. If it's your first exercise of the day, do as many sets as you feel necessary to properly warm up. We generally suggest two to four sets. If, for example, you are going to do dumbbell presses with fifty-pound dumbbells, warm up as light as twenty pounds and go through a full range of motion for fifteen to twenty repetitions. Then go to twenty or twenty-five and repeat, slow and controlled.

## WEIGHT-BASED EXERCISES

### Chest

#### Flat Bench Dumbbell Press

For this exercise, take a dumbbell in each hand and lie on your back on a flat bench. Bend at the elbows and press up, just as in a barbell bench press. With one exception: Turn your hands inward as you reach the top. Don't touch the dumbbells together. For working sets, do 12 to 15 repetitions.

#### Incline and Decline Dumbbell Press

These are merely slight variations of flat presses, using the pressing motion. Again with dumbbells, use either an incline or a decline bench. These offer another avenue of working the chest muscles. Particularly with the incline presses, you will want to make certain that you're not feeling any stress in your shoulders and collarbone area. If this is the case, adjust the incline until you feel it only in your chest.

## Biceps

### Dumbbell Curl

Simple techniques are often best. Almost everyone has seen this exercise. Just take a dumbbell in each hand at your side and, keeping your elbow in place, bring the dumbbell up as you turn your hand face up. Alternate sides.

When doing curls of any kind, make sure you're checking your ego at the door. All too often—and you'll notice this yourself by doing only minimal people-watching—guys try to impress fellow gym-goers by heaving massive amounts of weight on curls. Unfortunately, they're swinging their backs and putting themselves at serious risk while getting little to no benefit in the target muscles. Remember, fitness is about you. Pretend no one else is even working out around you, and always use proper form no matter how light or heavy you need to go with the weights.

### Hammer Curl

From the same position as in dumbbell curls, take a dumbbell in each hand and raise it toward your shoulder (again keeping your elbow still). The difference between these exercises is simply that with hammer curls, you don't twist your hand. This allows for another method of working the biceps as well as adding some work for the forearms.

You can add another variation to this exercise by sitting on an incline bench, allowing your arms to hang straight down, and starting from that hanging position.

## Triceps

### One-arm Triceps Extension

Take a dumbbell in one hand and raise your arm directly above your head. Bend at the elbow, drawing the dumbbell behind your head, and raise it back up to a near lockout (maintaining only a slight bend at the elbow). Alternate arms by set.

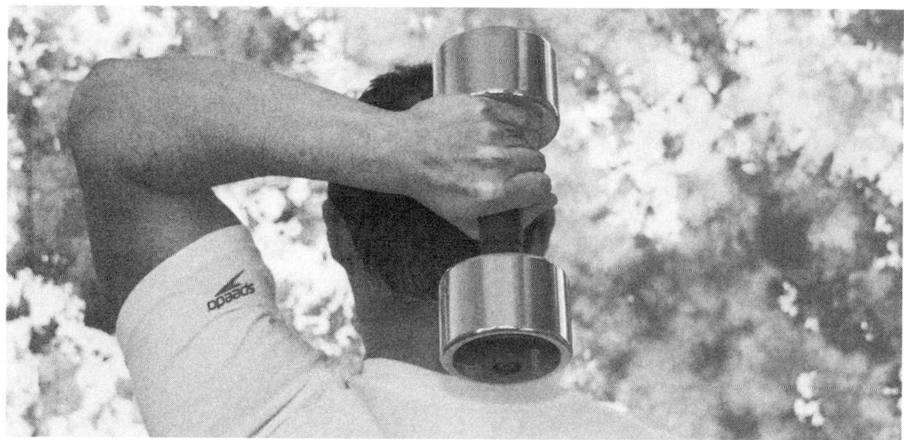

Keeping the elbow in one position allows the triceps to become fully involved in the exercise. Reach full extension and slowly return the weight behind your head.

### Dumbbell Kick-back

With a dumbbell in one hand, bend at the waist, keeping your back flat. Stagger your footing and place your free hand on something solid. With your arm in line with your body and your elbow close in, bend your arm into an L shape. Extend your arm directly back, twisting the wrist inward slightly as you reach full extension. Return to starting position. Alternate arms by set.

## Shoulders

### Shoulder Shrug

Stand up straight, keeping your head aligned with your spine and looking straight forward. With a dumbbell in each hand, at your sides, lift your shoulders as if you're trying to touch them to your ears. Pause momentarily at the top, then relax them back down. Don't roll your shoulders forward or back during the movement.

### Lateral Raise

Take a dumbbell in each hand, hold them at your sides (you'll need significantly lighter weights than you used for shrugs), and with your arms almost completely straight—except for a slight bend at the elbow—raise them up to just above shoulder level. Slowly bring them back to your sides.

## Back

### One-arm Row

Lean forward with your feet shoulder width apart and your right leg about two foot lengths behind the left in distance. With a dumbbell in your right hand, let the right arm hang straight down. Place your left hand on a solid, stable object in front of you, and pull the dumbbell in your right hand back to the side of your ribs. Alternate sides by set.

## Underhand Row

Similar to the one-arm row, stand with your feet in line and shoulder width apart, upper body just slightly forward. With a dumbbell in each hand, pull both back to the sides of your ribs.

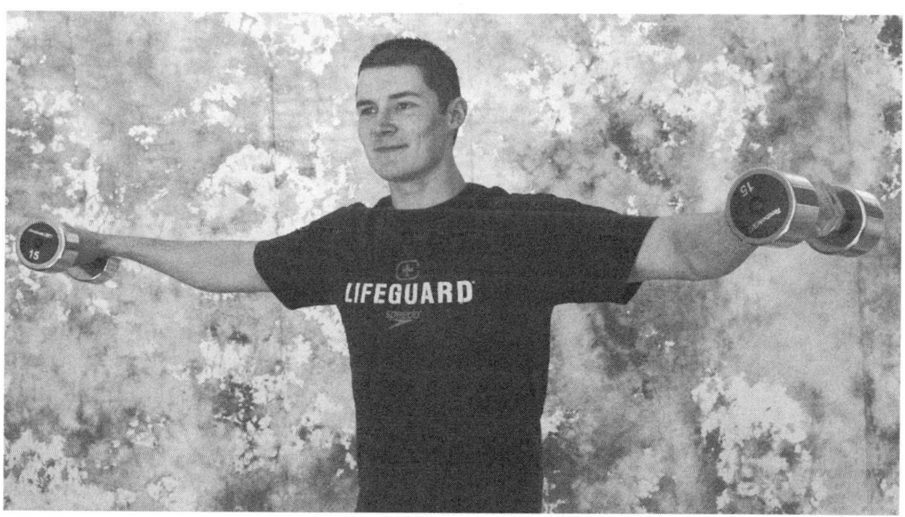


The deltoids are used in every swimming stroke, and lateral raises are one of the best ways to condition and strengthen them. Keep your arms only slightly bent and raise them to just above shoulder level.

# Legs

## Roman (stiff-legged) Dead Lift

These are done with a dumbbell in each hand, held at your side. With your knees straight (except for just a slight bend at the knee), lean forward. Keep the dumbbells in near the front of your legs—to keep the pressure off your lower back—and stop when you feel the flex in your hamstrings. Pause for a moment, then stand back up.

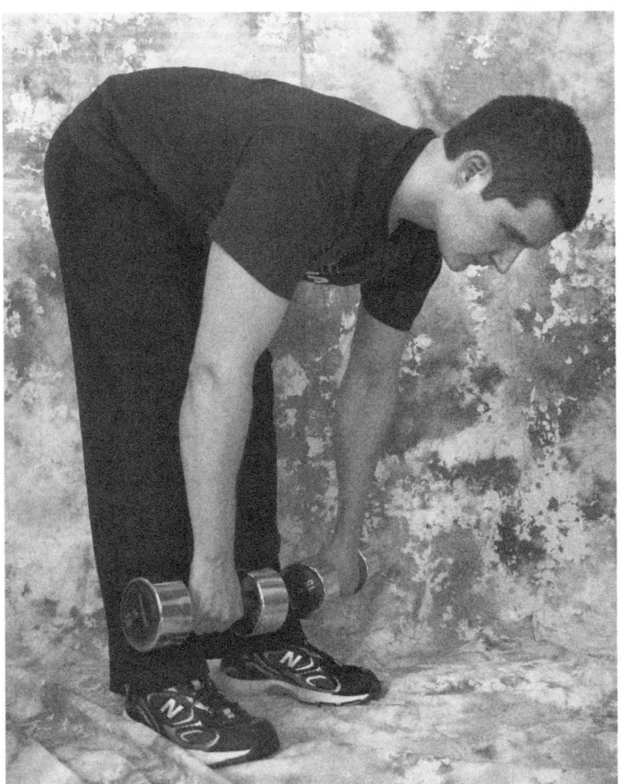

Strong legs can mean strong kicks. Stiff-legged dead lifts are done almost as the name indicates, but you do want to keep a slight bend at the knee to keep pressure off your lower back.

### Lunge

With a relatively light dumbbell in each hand, step as far forward as comfortable with your right leg and bend at the knees until your left knee is just above the ground. Your right shin should be vertical (flat up and down, at a 90-degree angle). Push back up from your right leg and return to your standing position. Alternate sides.

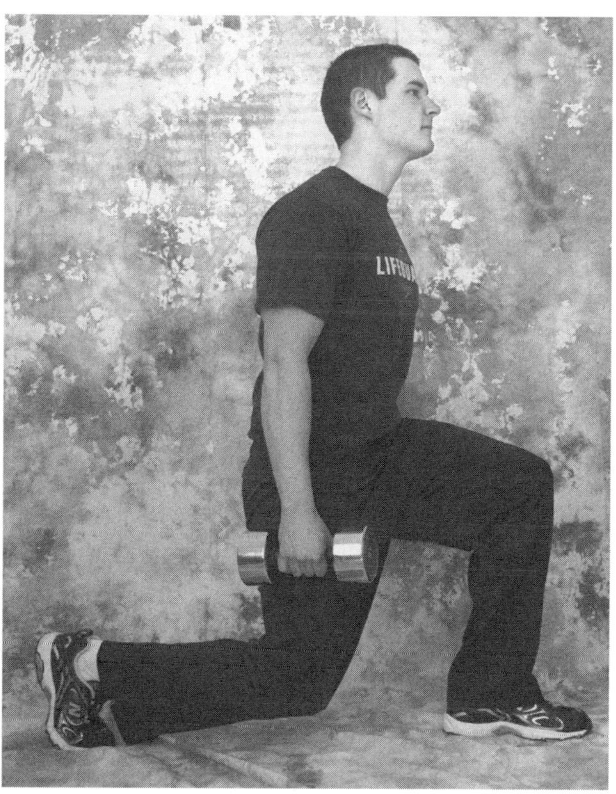

When you lunge forward, make sure your knee doesn't extend past your toes, and keep your back straight.

### Leg Extensions

This is a machine exercise where you sit, back flat against a pad, and place the lower portion of your shins against a pad. After setting a weight stack, usually with a pin, you extend your legs and feel set resistance. Do this exercise to work your quadriceps, pause at the extension of each set for just under one second, and return slowly to the starting position. These are generally done with both legs at once, but a great variation is to do them one leg at a time.

### Hamstring Curls

Another machine exercise; you lie facedown and place the pad just above your heels. Bending from the knee down, bring the pad toward your backside, and pause for just under one second when you're at the peak of contraction. Slowly return to starting position.

A note on speed: When lifting in these movements, use a smooth cadence in lifting the weight. Don't go fast enough that you begin to use momentum to get through the lift, but be sure you're not going "super" slow.

Many swimming and other athletic coaches incorrectly believe that lifts should be done extra slowly so that the muscle "burns" more, which is perceived to mean that muscular endurance is being built faster and that muscles are getting more gains from the prolonged workload.

However, a study in 2006 at the University of Connecticut found that extraslow repetitions actually decreased the amount of muscular strength built and the sustained muscular ability of muscle fibers when compared to normal-speed training with the same repetitions.

## PUSH/PULL CIRCUIT TRAINING

An advanced technique in the weight room that many athletes, swimmers especially, can benefit from is the introduction of specified circuit training into their programs.

We've seen a lot of coaches over the years just throw out a bunch of exercises and then tell their athletes to go for it, without stopping for rest, moving from exercise to exercise. Some are pretty experienced in what they're doing, others are less concerned with the muscle work and more with the cardiovascular conditioning, while still others seem to be doing it just because they can't think of anything else to have their athletes do, and they want them exercising more than just in the water.

Everything you do in your training should have an impact on your swimming. Even if you're not planning to race anytime in the near future, it only makes sense to do something that has a certain benefit to your overall progress. The most progress is made when you get the most out of an exercise, and if you go directly from doing fifty push-ups to doing fifty lunges, you're actually shortchanging yourself because energy expended in one area affects another, which prevents the legs from being fully worked.

One of the techniques that is beneficial for both sprinting and endurance athletes is a variation of circuit training called push/pull training. The goal with this is essentially to bring a great deal of blood into a specific area of the body for maximal wearing of the targeted muscles. Really, this sort of training is a hybrid. It isn't a full circuit of exercises, and not every movement is a push or a pull.

Because of the connotation the term "push/pull" provides of opposites, we're using that term only for simplicity.

This type of training is done with targeted movements and is used in conjunction with training muscle opposites. That is to say, if you're doing this to train your arms, you rotate from biceps to triceps. If for legs, from quadriceps to hamstrings. For lower core, from abdominals to the lower back. For the large muscles of the upper body, from chest to back.

There are both cardiovascular and strength benefits with this type of training because the weights are not intended to be extremely light, and you don't rest between sets.

Because there are only two parts to this, a front and a rear muscle, you're able to perform with quality weight to build muscle while keeping your heart rate up, causing the muscles to adapt in both weightbearing capacity and lasting ability.

To find the proper weight for you with this type of training, you'll adapt from your one-rep maximum lift (1RM). If you're not comfortable with finding your maximum lift, it's a much better idea to estimate rather than risk injury. Always use a spotter when doing heavy lifts as a safety precaution. If you do want to know your 1RM, warm up and attempt a certain weight. If you can do it, rest a few minutes and try a heavier weight.

An example of this for the biceps and triceps looks like this:

| | |
|---|---|
| Dumbbell biceps curls | 10–15 repetitions with 70% 1RM |
| Triceps machine pull-downs | 10–15 repetitions with 70% 1RM |
| Rest 30 seconds | |
| Dumbbell biceps curls | 8–12 repetitions with 70% 1RM |
| Triceps machine pull-downs | 8–12 repetitions with 70% 1RM |

Rest 15 seconds

| | |
|---|---|
| Dumbbell biceps curls | 6–10 repetitions with 70% 1RM |
| Triceps machine pull-downs | 6–10 repetitions with 70% 1RM |

The reason the rep schemes vary by four to five repetitions each set is because based on your conditioning level you may be able to do more on a certain exercise than others, and you never want to shortchange yourself. As with any sort of weight training, if you pick up a weight with the determination that, for example, eight reps should be hard, don't stop just because you're at eight if you could do more. Finish when your muscles have been thoroughly used, and adjust the weight appropriately for the next set.

If you follow through the repeats in the example, your arms should be very tired. Because of the strain, we suggest taking on this type of workload at the beginning of your workout, after a solid warm-up. You can make a complete workout for those muscle groups by going through that routine, resting for two to five minutes, and then repeating it in the opposite order (triceps, then biceps).

Now that you have an idea of how this works, we'll change it up just slightly by showing you a pair for the quadriceps and hamstrings, and explain the differences you'll see right away.

| | |
|---|---|
| Leg extensions | 16–20 repetitions with 70% 1RM |
| Hamstring curls | 16–20 repetitions with 70% 1RM |
| Rest 45 seconds | |
| Leg extensions | 12–15 repetitions with 70% 1RM |
| Hamstring curls | 12–15 repetitions with 70% 1RM |
| Rest 30 seconds | |

| | |
|---|---|
| Leg extensions | 8–12 repetitions with 70% 1RM |
| Hamstring curls | 8–12 repetitions with 70% 1RM |

Here you've seen an opposites routine (push/pull variation) with larger muscle groups, and it started out with a higher number of repetitions. Why?

We changed our training based on some interesting research from the University of Connecticut. Researchers there found that at submaximal intensities, study participants were able to complete more repetitions of an exercise based on the amount of muscle mass in a given area of the body. In their test, repetition capacity was higher across the board with the squat—large muscles—as compared to biceps curls—small muscles. This was the same for trained and untrained participants.

After reading this a couple of years ago, we tried it out, found the results to be very impressive, and have utilized varied rep schemes ever since to great benefit. Once you try it, you'll see that this, too, is another example of different volume requirements for different muscles.

Push/pull and opposites training are a great way to train a given area of the body. Give them a try and feel free to mix them into your program as another exciting training method that will help break up the monotony of straight-set work. Try adding it in every other week or so.

## WEIGHT-FREE EXERCISES

For some people, weights aren't feasible. Either cost or comfort can play a part. In any case, you can still supplement your swim training with any land exercise, weight-free.

### Chest

#### Incline and Decline Push-up

Similarly to the variations on dumbbell presses from a bench, you can get a workout by just elevating either your arms or your feet. These can be done as easily as placing your feet up on a couch and going through the same push-up motion. Likewise, you can find a solid elevated platform, like a sitting bench, place your hands on its edge, and push up from that position.

### Triceps

#### Triceps Dip

Use a step bench for this exercise. Sit down on the floor next to it and place your hands over the edges with the palms of your hands flat on the surface. Extend your legs out straight until you're far enough away that your backside can clear the bench. Bend at the elbows until your triceps are flat (your butt should be just slightly off the bench or ground at this point), then push yourself up.

## Back

### Lower Back Bend

Standing straight up, lock your fingers behind your head and bend forward at the waist, then return to your starting position. Make sure you have only a slight bend in your knees.

### Half Bridge

Lie on your back with your knees bent and the bottoms of your feet planted firmly on the ground. Push from your legs to bring your lower back off the ground and lift your hips as high as possible. Pause at the peak, then return to the ground. This will help strengthen your lower back and is best done in high repetitions.

## Abdominals

In addition to the classic crunches and sit-ups, there are a couple of other beneficial exercises you can do for your frontal core.

### Leg Lift

Lying flat on your back with your hands underneath your butt, start with your heels about four inches off the ground. Raise your legs together as high as you can while maintaining contraction—if you feel your abdominal muscles relax, you've gone too far. Return to the starting position.

### Knee Bend

From the same starting position as leg lifts, bend at the knees and pull them back toward your chest. Return to the starting position. Pause for a moment before repeating.

### Elbow Lift

Get into a push-up position, but rather than holding yourself up on your hands, place your elbows and forearms on the ground and keep your back flat. Hold this position for a set amount of time—depending on what's difficult for you—and do several repeats of that time. Perhaps one minute on, one minute of rest, four times over.

## Legs

### Lunge

Just as with weights but with your hands on your hips instead, follow the same routine as outlined under the weight-based exercises.

### Body Weight Squat

Stand with your legs shoulder width apart and place your hands either on your hips or behind your head. Squat down until your quadriceps—your upper thigh—become flat, and return to standing straight up.

### Calf Raise

Stand on a step bench with your heels hanging off the edge. Push from the balls of your feet until you are as tall as possible, then slowly return to below platform level. Pause at the bottom—you should feel your calves stretch.

### Hip Raise

Lie on your left side and prop yourself up on your left elbow. With your toes pointing toward the wall you're facing, raise your right leg as high as possible, pause at its peak, and bring it back down. Alternate sides.

## PUTTING TOGETHER A ROUTINE

It would be impossible for one workout to suit everyone. With each body being so different and strength changing from person to person, there's no one-size-fits-all workout. But there are some general guidelines you can use to put together just the right program for your own body.

The larger body parts need higher-volume work than do smaller parts. Below are suggested numbers for total sets around the body per workout:

| Body Part | Sets |
|---|---|
| Chest | 10 |
| Biceps | 6 |
| Triceps | 6 |
| Shoulders | 8 |
| Back | 10 |
| Quads | 8 |
| Hamstrings | 8 |
| Calves | 10 |

Remember, these are just suggestions for a new trainer. You'll notice that the bigger body parts are suggested to be worked between eight and ten sets each week (not per exercise), with smaller muscle groups at six. Calves are unique in that, while small, they are in constant use every day, so they need additional work.

It's also important to keep in mind that these numbers aren't set in stone. They can be adjusted depending on your recovery speed, experience, and goals.

If you're not sore after a workout, that doesn't necessarily mean you need more volume. You may just need more intensity. Always warm up, but don't be afraid to go heavy as long as your form is good. And remember that heavy is relative; there is no set number that qualifies as heavy. If ten-pound curls are difficult, they're heavy for you. Always keep form in mind. Any set where your form is sacrificed right away due to a heavier weight is *too heavy*.

Sets should range between fifteen and twenty reps for beginners. When you're not comfortable using heavy weights, it can lead to injury. Higher reps will still provide solid results for a new trainer. Once you're comfortable with form, you can advance to heavier weights and slightly fewer reps.

Lower reps with relative heavy weight will cause a greater deal of muscle growth than higher-repetition, relatively lighter weight resistance exercise. But keep in mind that swimming is essentially a constant resistance exercise, and if you're trying to become a faster swimmer—which would mean you need to mimic the water, as we said earlier—you need to be doing more sets to re-create the type of stress.

Competitive and fitness swimmers alike need to be functional and efficient in the water. For the competitive swimmer it's all about speed, and for the fitness swimmer it's about having the physical capacity to carry out the effort necessary in the pool to achieve goals. In either case, you're in need of not only strength but also muscular endurance.

If you're looking to build muscular endurance after a few months of dryland training experience, keep your repetitions between twelve and fifteen and reduce rest between sets to fifteen to forty-five seconds. Again, you're mimicking pool training. Swimmers develop their endurance in the water by reducing recovery time between sets of substantial effort, and that principle works on solid ground, too.

If strength is your goal, stick to sets in the six-to-ten-repetition range.

One important exception to this rule is that if you're a training competitive swimmer, and a sprinter in particular, you can benefit from some of the heavier-weight, lower-repetition "explosive" weight training. In fact, you can reduce your reps down to as low as four and five for basic compound exercises on special sets, done one to two times weekly. If you're doing so, be sure it's a weight that lets you explode into a positive contraction. Don't use a weight so heavy that you struggle from the moment you lift it off the rack or the bar.

It's going to be up to you and your knowledge of your own body to determine the type of training you need at any given time. We feel strongly that everyone who is new to dryland training should start off light and with a higher number of repetitions per set for safety, but after that, you're able to decide the course you'd like to take.

It's impossible to build muscular endurance for muscle you don't have. If in the past your nutrition hasn't been the best or your effort hasn't quite been there to make strides with your physique, then it's likely you'll want to employ a few more sets of lifts designed to pack on some muscle. Mix up your workouts and develop a foundation to work from.

On the other end we have the people who either put on muscle very easily or have trained for years to develop a good core of size and strength. If this is you, the goal should be to become efficient. You'll need to train your muscles to put up with longer bouts of oxygen deprivation to get you through your water workouts. In these cases, use good, strict form, and keep your reps higher.

## THE BENEFIT OF FAILURE

While you don't want to employ it in every single set, going to failure—the point where you're physically unable to complete another rep—is a quality technique to ensure the working of all your

Olympian Tip **The Importance of Strength Training**

***Gary Hall Jr.—***
***ten-time medalist, 1996 Atlanta, 2000 Sydney, 2004 Athens Olympics***

Strength training is necessary, especially after you mature. Strength training for someone who is young and developing is less important, and the chance of injury is greater. When training for the Olympics, I swim a lot. But I spend as much, if not more, time training out of the pool. Sprint freestyle is a power sport. You can get more power in the weight room.

muscle fibers for not just strength but also endurance. This applies in both the weight room and the pool.

Think about it; if you swam a 100-yard freestyle race every single day but slowed down as soon as it started to get hard, how quickly do you think you would improve? Likewise, what if every day you pushed through the pain and kept trying even when your body wanted to give up? Sometimes you just have to make the body do things it doesn't want to do.

15

# Stretching

*Stretching is, overall,* one of the most important physical activities that people can do. Unfortunately, most neglect this, and not only do their athletic abilities suffer, but so does the comfort of their daily life.

If you think about it, tight muscles restrict blood flow and increase the risk of injury. They're uncomfortable when sitting, standing, and even moving around. People who live sedentary lives are generally stiffer, less flexible, more lethargic, and are at a greater risk of injury than their active peers. These things can be improved just by stretching regularly, and as a result the muscles will recover better from other workouts, you will feel more energetic, and you will receive all sorts of other benefits.

So here are some stretches you should do every day—they take only about fifteen to twenty minutes combined—and it's a great start to getting in shape and potentially preventing injury.

## WARM-UP

First off, always start by warming up. Stretching without a little warm-up can be a bad idea. You don't want to jump right into one of your workout sets, but if you're getting ready for a pool workout, get in and swim an easy few laps. Stop for a minute or two, then repeat. Do four or five repetitions of that, hop out, do your stretches, and then return to the water.

If you're on dry land, do some squats just standing in place; do about ten or fifteen, rest for a few seconds, do another fifteen or twenty. Repeat that until you feel warm, and you're done with your lower half.

You'll need to also do some arm raises: Just lift your arms out to your sides slowly, just to above shoulder height, then lower them. Fifteen or twenty is great. Then drop down, do ten push-ups, rest for up to a minute, do ten or fifteen more, and you're good to go from top to bottom.

Naturally, your warm-up should vary depending on your physical abilities. If twenty push-ups is your absolute limit already, warming up with that many repetitions isn't a good idea. Warming up isn't about pushing the limits; just do what feels good.

For the following stretches, hold each one for at least 15 seconds, and be sure to work both sides.

## CHEST

Start with some chest stretches. Standing with feet shoulder width apart, place an arm flat on the wall, horizontally at shoulder level, and slowly rotate away from it. Repeat on the other side. After you've done both sides, return to the first side you stretched, and rotate your hand; just turn the hand until your thumb and first finger are on the wall instead of your palm. This slight variation is a stretch for your arm in addition to your front deltoid and chest. Again, as with all individual stretches, do both sides. Yet another variant of this chest-stretching position is to simply bend your arm on the wall at the elbow, so that your fingers point upward.

## TRICEPS

To stretch your triceps, raise one arm straight up, bend at the elbow so your hand ends up behind your head and a bit down your back, and use your other arm to gently pull back on the elbow.

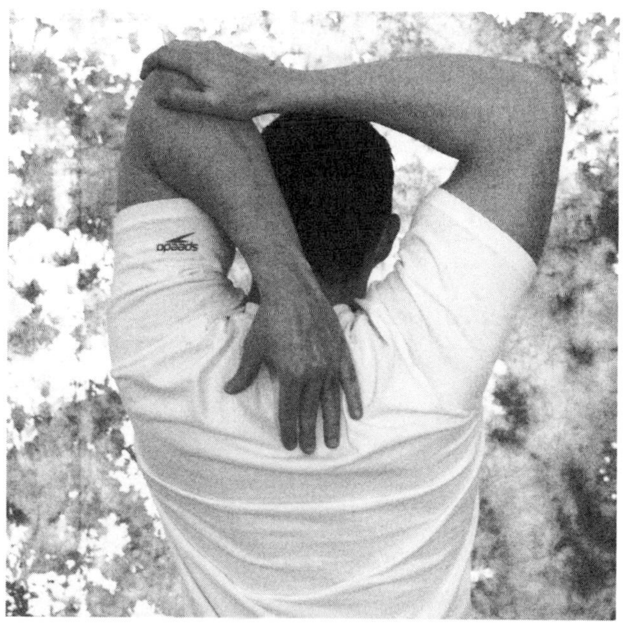


When you pull back on your elbow, always start slowly and never do more than is comfortable.

## FOREARMS

Stretch your forearms by using one hand to push back the flat fingers of the other (again, go slowly).

## BACK

To stretch your lats and core, do a "streamline" with your arms and keep your legs shoulder width apart. Raise both of your arms straight up, have your hands flat and overlapping, and push your biceps over your ears. Hold this for a few seconds, then try to (figuratively) touch your fingertips to the ceiling. Then, slowly and gently, lean to either side. When you bring your arms down after you finish this stretch, do so slowly.

Lie on the ground on your back, arms straight out and flat on the ground, and bring your right leg over to the left side of your body, bent at the knee. Repeat on the other side.

## GROIN

Stretch your groin by standing with your feet just comfortably outside shoulder width, and lean your hips in either direction. Be sure to keep your feet flat and not lean into your ankles.

## HIPS

To stretch your hips, sit on the floor, cross one leg over the other, and bend at the knee until that foot is flat on the ground. Rotate your torso in the direction of the leg you're bending, and lightly press against the side of the leg to stretch the hip.

Sitting with your legs straight out, cross one leg over the other and bend that leg at the knee. Place your foot flat, and rotate to the side at the bent knee while gently pulling on your knee to the foot side.

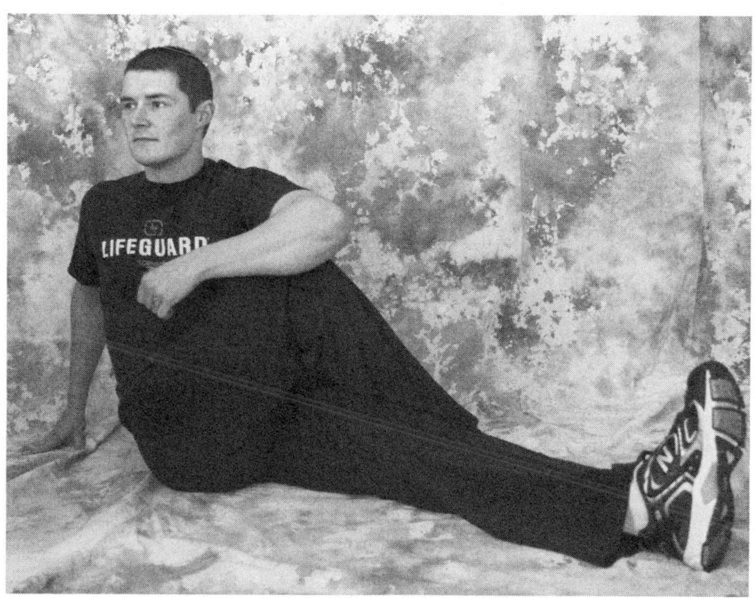


Hip flexibility is especially beneficial in breaststroke. Slowly press against your leg until you feel the stretch, then pause. Push farther only if it is comfortable to do so.

## QUADS

To stretch your quads, place one hand on a wall for stability (if necessary), and use the other to pull that same side's foot up to your backside. Keep the knee of the leg you're stretching in line (up and down) with the knee of the leg you're still standing on.

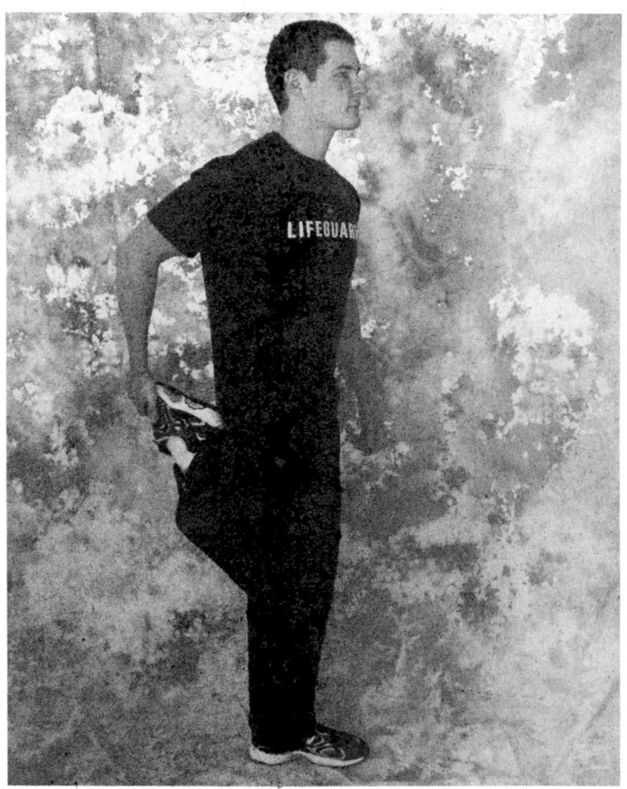


Be sure to breathe out and relax while stretching to make sure your muscles can extend. If you're tense, it's more difficult to stretch properly.

From your knees, point your toes behind you so that the tops of your feet are on the ground. Using your hands for balance, slowly lean backward as if you were trying to lie on top of your feet.

The previous stretch can also be done one leg at a time. Simply place the opposite leg out straight in front of you.

## HAMSTRINGS

For your hamstrings, just stand straight, feet together, with a slight bend in the knees, and try to put your hands on the floor. Be sure not to bounce, and move slowly as you proceed.

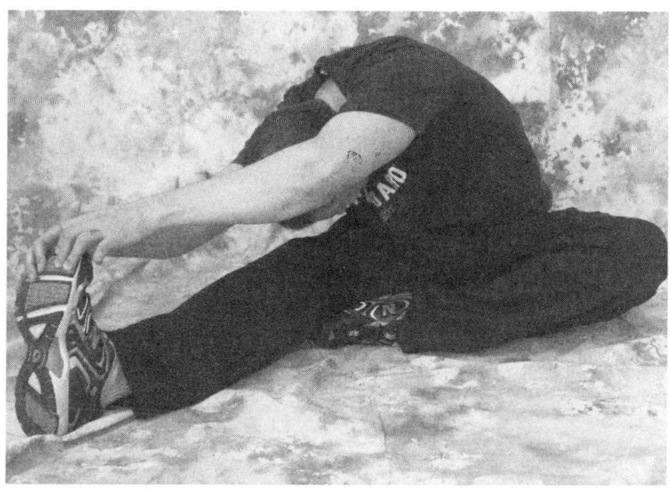

This stretch will work your back as well as your hamstrings. Breathe out and relax as you lean forward, and be careful not to bounce back and forth. Relax into the stretch.

While sitting on the floor, extend one leg fully outward and pull the other foot in so the bottom touches the inside of the thigh of your opposite leg. Slowly reach with both arms toward the toes of the extended leg, grabbing your toes if you can.

## CALVES

For your calves, stand in front of a wall and just lift the ball of your foot onto it while keeping your heel down. Gently lean into it and you'll feel it. Do this one leg at a time.

There are dozens of stretches you can do, so pick and choose your favorites. They may not all be comfortable at first, but keep in mind how good they can be for you. When done properly, they can increase performance, prevent injury, enhance recovery, and simply make you feel better all day long.

16

# Medicine Ball Training

One of the more versatile dryland exercise methods you can incorporate into your training is the use of a medicine ball. These look like an average basketball but are of varied sizes (smaller or larger depending on the weight). Get one that also bounces at your local sports store, and you have a simple tool that can be used almost anywhere for a great workout. Here are some basic exercises.

## CHEST

### Chest Pass

This isn't an exercise you want to do at home, but this is a variation of the partner version of the exercise. When you're by yourself, find a solid wall (brick or concrete) and face it. Stand close enough that you can quickly bounce the ball off the wall. Use small tosses and continually bounce the ball off the wall, catch it, and repeat. Use high repetitions in this as you don't want to use a weight so heavy that you harm your wrists by catching it.

## ARMS

### Triceps Raises

Stand up straight with correct posture (back straight, head in line) and hold a medicine ball tightly on each side. Raise your arms straight up above your head, then bend at the elbows to bring the ball behind your head. After pausing in this position, return to the start position. For proper form, make sure the elbows stay in place. A very common mistake with this exercise is to let the elbows flare out.

### Biceps Curls

Probably the simplest of all medicine ball exercises; you simply place a medicine ball in the palm of your hand, with your palm facing upward. Extend your arm straight down with your wrist bent just enough to maintain your hold on the ball, then bend at the elbow to curl the ball upward. Pause at peak contraction, then return to the starting position.

### Front Raise

Hold a medicine ball tightly by its sides with your arms straight, in a standing position. Start with the medicine ball in front of your legs and raise your arms up slowly to bring the ball in line with your face. Pause at that point before returning to the starting position.

## LOWER BACK BENDS

In doing this exercise, be sure to use a relatively light medicine ball to ensure safety.

Hold a medicine ball tight against your chest while standing straight up. With only a slight bend in the knees, bend over at the waist until your back is flat, pause, and return to starting position.

## ABDOMINALS

### Oblique Twist

These are done by simply standing up tall with good posture and holding a medicine ball against your body at the top of your abs. Twist the upper half of your body as far as you comfortably can to one side, pause, and twist over to the other side.

### Crunch

These are well known to everyone but can be enhanced by holding a medicine ball to your chest while going through the movement. To increase the difficulty of this exercise, while your abs are contracted at the peak of your crunch, pause for one or two seconds before returning to the starting position.

### Leg Raise

These are done by lying on the ground with your legs fully extended and your arms fully extended so that you're as long as possible. Hold the medicine ball (a light one for safety) tightly between your hands.

Bend your body into a V shape by lifting your legs upward as your upper body moves forward to meet them. Try to touch the ball (keeping your arms straight) to your toes before returning to the starting position.

### Leg Raise with a Pass

This is a more difficult variation of the leg raise exercise. It is done the same way, except that at peak contraction (when you're in the V shape) you place the ball between your feet and return to the starting position with the medicine ball held by your ankles instead of your hands. On the next rep, you trade it back to your hands and repeat the whole process.

## LEGS

### Squat

Squats are taken to a whole new level with the addition of a medicine ball. For squats, simply hold the medicine ball to your chest and go through the motions for a weighted version of a great movement.

### Lunge

For lunges, you can hold the medicine ball at your chest as well, or if that alters your balance, you can hold it with both hands behind your neck.

### Riding Stance

With your feet about two inches on either side past shoulder width apart, bend at the knees so that both quadriceps are flat. This alone is a great endurance exercise, but it becomes quite a bit more difficult when you're holding a medicine ball. Hold it at your chest (just under your chin), or to stress your deltoid muscles as well, hold it straight out in front of you with your arms.

As you can tell, there's little that can't be done with a simple medicine ball. There's so much you can do to improve your fitness level, even if the weight isn't heavy enough to build extremely large muscles (if that's not your goal, then it's not even an issue).

If there was only one piece of exercise equipment you could have, this would be it. Try it out and see for yourself; use it in conjunction with other dryland activities or on its own. The choice is yours! If you want to keep things mixed up, one way to do so is to alternate dryland training techniques by week. Perhaps three weeks in the gym, one or two doing medicine ball work, and repeat.

# 17

# Cross-Training

If it seems to you as though swimming is too good to be true, that's understandable. For all the benefits of exercising in the water, the lack of side effects makes it seem as if there must be a catch! Luckily, it's reality that swimming can help you live longer and healthier. In fact, despite all the benefits already covered, it gets better.

Swimming is one of the best activities you can perform to improve your performance in other sports. It's obvious how swimming can benefit one's water polo skills, but even land-based athletes benefit greatly from beginning an intelligent aquatic training program.

A common misconception about cross-training is that you need to do a similar activity—tennis or golf for baseball, running for football, things that mimic what your primary sport involves. While those types of sports are certainly going to benefit your main athletic pursuits, you could very well get even better results by doing something that, on the surface, has little to do with your sport. For almost every sport, swimming is about as far away as you can get. Or, at least, it would seem that way.

On the most basic level, every sport uses a variety of muscles; some more than others. Running is a great example of a sport where a specific group of muscles is obviously more involved. In fact, most runners don't train their upper body at all because of the added weight and drag caused by additional mass. With this restriction in mind, there are far fewer choices for cross-training in football, for example, which uses all major muscle groups.

In any case, though, no matter what restrictions are in place, an athlete can use swimming to cross-train. With the repetitive motions of some sports creating a higher likelihood of injury, swimming can not only help keep the body in shape while giving it a breather from its normal wear and tear, it can further enhance your cardiovascular system, improve your muscular endurance, and strengthen both your major muscle groups and the smaller, stabilizing muscles. Here is a look at some accompanying sets and training protocols to increase your ability in other sports.

## UPPER-BODY SPORTS

A huge variety of athletes can benefit from an enhanced form of upper-body musculature. And while swimming is a repetitive action, using the same muscles repeatedly, there are also several forms

| Stroke | Primary Upper-Body Muscle(s) Worked |
|---|---|
| Backstroke | Back, triceps, shoulders |
| Breaststroke | Chest, biceps, lower back |
| Butterfly | Shoulders, triceps, abs |
| Freestyle | Triceps, shoulders, back |

of swimming that allow you to concentrate on working particular upper-body muscles. A great aid in isolating muscle groups is the use of a pull buoy, because you don't have to worry about keeping your hips up.

Every stroke obviously uses many more muscles than just listed, but these are muscles that can be easily targeted by swimming that particular stroke.

For example, to target your deltoids and trapezius muscles, do a butterfly pull one arm at a time, alternating by five strokes. Swim with one arm ahead and the other arm taking five strokes, then switch. By breathing to the side and using a buoy you'll increase the length for which you can pull.

When you do this, don't use a kick-out or, for breaststroke, a pull-out. While those are great techniques that deserve plenty of practice, this is targeted training and you're focusing on specific muscle groups; if you use up a quarter of the pool before going into your stroke, you're using up more oxygen underwater and targeting the focus muscles less.

For this type of targeted training, use longer distances. Try sets of 100- to 200-yard swims to ensure you're really fatiguing the muscles, as with a buoy you can go a lot farther than if you were fully swimming.

Also make sure you're placing extreme emphasis on making your pull long and using a full range of motion. If you're using only half strokes or not extending fully, you're not activating all potential muscle fibers. If you're getting long on the recovery, be just as long on the finish. If in freestyle, for instance, you're not fully extending your arm and finishing past your hips, you are not using your triceps as much as you could be.

It's important to note that you want to have a solid foundation of technique before doing stroke-specific muscle work. That isn't to say you won't get muscular strength and endurance benefits while you're perfecting your technique, because you will, but rather than going right after those 200-yard swims, take the time and make sure you have a great foundation. Improper technique being repeated in this type of work will not only assist in developing bad habits, but it will also reduce the gains from the exercise.

It would be impossible to list specific cross-training workouts for every sport. Luckily, we don't have to, because athletics share common necessities in endurance, sprinting, and lactate threshold training.

The following are some good sets based on your goals. After you get the hang of how they're tailored—which we will explain with details in each set—you'll be able to develop some of your own. After all, the *Get Wet, Get Fit* ideology is based around individual enjoyment of the sport and an understanding of what you're doing and why you're doing it. There's nothing quite like creating your own workout with a purpose, completing it in its entirety, and feeling the benefits from it in the end.

If you're comfortable in the water, you can do these sets and gain from them. They aren't on a send-off (set times to finish) but instead are based on your own abilities and adjusting your effort levels. Because swimming taxes the body on aerobic and anaerobic fronts, you will be adjusting your efforts from time to time.

## LEG-INTENSE SPORTS

### Running

Running is about as intense as you can get when it comes to giving your legs a pounding. Obviously, runners, like any other athletes, want to get better. Some runners, no doubt, don't think swimming will do much for them. So if taking the word of their fellow athletes isn't good enough, how about an authority on the sport? Runners World.com, the online destination for *Runner's World* magazine fans, answered the question "Does lap swimming have any cross-training value for running?" The answer, of course, is that it certainly does. The contributor answering the question explained that the "beauty of swimming is that it helps you maintain cardiorespiratory fitness while simultaneously strengthening and soothing your body." In addition, it was suggested that after a hard day on the track, a runner should get in the pool to aid recovery.

According to State of the Art Marathon Training (www.marathontraining.com), a site dedicated to helping people prepare for and complete marathons, swimming is one of the best cross-training activities available. The site describes its benefits as muscular strength and endurance and increased flexibility. Running is very specific in terms of the muscles worked during the activity. With each step, the same muscles and joints are "abused" during warm-up, cool-down, training, and racing. That's one of the things that separates running from other sports, and one of the reasons swimming is so beneficial for it.

Training in the water works muscles that aren't used or as heavily relied on when going around the track. It can benefit you in other areas, too, such as your breathing.

In any endurance sport, oxygen consumption is vital. When swimming, you follow a specific pattern. Your body can't simply act and take in air whenever you'd like, as it can when you're running. You have to follow a pattern that includes a period when taking in air isn't possible (whenever your head is submerged beneath the surface). This lung control helps your body use oxygen more efficiently, which can be transferred to your running.

Further strengthening your legs through the motions of swim kicking is a great tool to enhance your running. For this, we'll focus on flutter kicking, as you would use when swimming freestyle or backstroke. This kick is the most effective for targeting your quadriceps and hamstrings. Additionally, we'll discuss breaststroke kicking, which will involve your hips more.

## Olympian Tip Importance of Kick Training

***Gabe Woodward—***
***bronze medalist, 2004 Athens Olympics***

The legs are the engine that powers the boat. In order to swim your fastest you must have your legs in amazing condition. For sprinters, this means lots of sprint kicking so that you can swim the race and have your legs running at full throttle the entire time without having to think about them. It's such a bummer when your legs tighten up in a sprint because they aren't in top condition. However, it's fantastic when you near the end of your race and feel your legs still going full throttle!

## Training Sets for Your Legs: Flutter Kicking

Start with an alternating pattern of 20 flutter kicks easy (each leg movement counts as 1) followed by 10 fast. Repeat for 3 sets of 50-yard repetitions, resting 1 minute between.

### Increasing Difficulty

If you want to further the challenge and increase results, you can do so in a variety of ways. First, cut down on your rest. This challenges your muscles and your body to act with less oxygen and less recovery. Second, you can reduce the number of easy kicks or increase the fast kicks, or both. Last, you can extend the set's duration.

### Set to Failure

It is important that you do the following only once in a great while, as you don't want it to significantly alter your abilities out of the pool: Instead of going with preconceived sets for a given length, you can employ a technique used by many athletes in the weight room: You can go to failure, which is to say you simply go until you can't go anymore. In this case, you finish the set only after you are no longer able to complete the proper number of fast kicks. Many people find kicking sets difficult because the legs quickly begin to "burn," and they give up. Despite this feeling, though, most people can go significantly further. If you want to challenge yourself and really see where you stand, give this set a shot.

## BREASTSTROKE KICKING

You can do the same types of sets for breaststroke kicking, which will allow further refinement for the muscles in the hips and glutes. Of course, there are other variations you can do with breaststroke kicking to increase the difficulty.

Kickboard Resistance: Hold a kickboard out in front of you vertically in the water. This creates a literal wall in front of you, which your kick has to overpower to move forward.

When training your legs with breaststroke kicking, make sure you're strict with your movement. If you separate your knees past the normal suggested width, you'll take the focus away from the hips.

### Leg-intense sports

Basketball players and others can gain a lot of benefits from breaststroke kicking. Because of the intense hip training, vertical leaps can largely be improved. Be sure to train your legs with strong sets of breaststroke kicking, and stretch the muscles worked.

## MEASURING YOUR HEART RATE

Your maximum heart rate is roughly 220 minus your age. So for a twenty-year-old, his/her maximum is 200.

For the following sets you'll need to know how to take your heart rate so you can reach and maintain the percentage given. To do so, all you have to do is use the index and middle fingers of one hand to find the pulse in your wrist or your neck (just to the side of your throat). Count the beats for six seconds, then multiply by ten, or count for ten seconds and multiply by six.

Whenever you're exercising, knowing your HR is good information.

Between sets, or during your rest periods, take your heart rate and determine if you need to increase or decrease your efforts.

## ENDURANCE TRAINING

Your entire goal is to perform at a high level for a longer period of time. Technique isn't enough in athletic events that last; you have to have the lung capacity and muscular capabilities to keep going when everyone else wants to quit. If that sounds like your sport, give these workouts a shot.

As always, be sure to get a good warm-up in prior to commencing these sets.

### Set #1

This set gives you aerobic benefits from longer swims, broken every 200 or 400 yards. Your heart rate stays elevated—a must—because of the relatively short rest periods.

2 x 200 freestyle @ 65% :15R

Two freestyle swims, 200 yards each (2 x 200) at an effort that equals 65% of your maximal heart rate (@ 65%) on fifteen seconds rest between swims (:15R)

3 x 400 freestyle @ 75% :20R

## Set #2

You don't have to swim huge amounts of yards in a row to gain endurance benefits. While distance is a must, it can be broken. This set takes advantage of building into short swims with very little rest.

20 x 25 freestyle @ 70% :5R

15 x 50 freestyle @ 70% :5R

15 x 50 @ 75% :10R

Odd—backstroke

Even—freestyle

## Set #3

Except for the most die-hard swimmers, swimming the same stroke for miles on end can get boring. Endurance training, luckily, doesn't have to get stale. You can mix it up and swim your favorite stroke as long as you keep your effort within the levels.

5 x 100 IM (by 25) @75 % :15R

4 x 150 alternate freestyle, favorite stroke by 50 @ 70% :15R

4 x 200 freestyle, every third length favorite stroke @70% :15R

# SPRINT TRAINING

## Set #1

So you're a sprinter, right? You don't necessarily enjoy miles of yardage, and you don't necessarily need it. The goal in sprint training is intensity, absolute full-on intensity. Get it up, and keep it up, for short periods of maximal effort. If you want to be a great sprinter, teach your body how to sprint. The best way is simply to do it.

1 x 100 freestyle @ 80% 3:30R

1 x 100 IM @ 100% 4:00R

2 x 50 freestyle @ 80% 1:30R

1 x 50 freestyle @ 100% 2:00R

**2 rounds**

### Set #2

Sprinting builds your anaerobic abilities over that which you developed during aerobic training. Between sprints you want to allow your body enough time to break down and pass as much lactate (an ester of lactic acid) as possible. The sooner it goes, the better you will feel as lactate causes that burn you feel during tough training. That being said, enjoy the rest because if you've done the set right, you'll have certainly earned it.

5 x 50 freestyle @ 95% 1:30R

3 x 50 favorite stroke except freestyle@ 95% 1:30R

3 x 100 freestyle, second and fourth lengths your choice of stroke @ 95% 3:00R

## LACTATE THRESHOLD TRAINING

You may be what we swimmers call a "middle-distance" athlete. You need more than sprinting ability, because your race demands more to be successful, but you don't tap into your maximal aerobic capacity because the race doesn't take you there. You're in need of lactate threshold training, which teaches your body to hold on to its maximal performance abilities for longer than it was intended to.

That, in all honesty, takes a lot of guts to train for properly. Each of these sets should be performed at full intensity. We won't denote percentages here because they're all the same: everything you've got!

### Set #1

Unlike in sprinting, you can't rest as long between sets because you have to get used to performing with pain. Not injury pain, of course, but the pain that develops when lactic acid builds up. Just as in this set.

All freestyle

8 x 25 :10R

4 x 50 :10R

3 x 75 :15R

2 x 100 :20R

You'll notice that these sets only gently increase rest periods as the distance increases each length. You'll get tired, and that's the point. When you "hit the wall," so to speak, it's after that point—as you keep going—that your body begins to learn what you want it to know and retain.

## Set #2

Short and intense. With lactate threshold training it isn't the feel right away, it's what develops and how you handle it. This training develops the ability to give all of your effort over and over.

12 x 25 IM :10R

10 x 25 freestyle :5R

Rest one minute

12 x 25 IM :10R

# 18

# Rehabilitation

*Swimming can improve* the quality of your life, improve your athletic skills for other sports, and help reduce the likelihood of injury in land-based activities. But if you do end up injured—on the job or on the field, court, or track—the pool may still be the very best place for you to heal.

Over the years, the water has been the most-chosen method of getting people back to activity after all kinds of physical ailments, ranging anywhere from broken bones to heart attacks. The reason for this is because swimming offers a free range of motion, puts no excessive strain on the body as weight training does, and allows you to progress at your own pace. Becoming a better swimmer, like recovering from an injury, takes time and effort. Luckily, being in the water can achieve both simultaneously.

## SWIMMING BACK TO HEALTH

Is swimming right for your injury? It probably is. The activity is low impact, and the resistance of the water provides great cardiovascular exercise as well as a wonderful method to maintain and build strength.

A few points are necessary before deciding that swimming is right for your personal needs in rehabilitation. The first step is to see a doctor to see if he recommends it and be sure that swimming isn't going to further injure you. Also, see if he has specific guidelines for what you should and should not be doing in the pool. If you have a particularly bad shoulder injury, for instance, freestyle may not be for you. Depending on where the tear or stretch is, butterfly might be out of the question. Generally, there's something for everyone in the water, but be sure to avoid anything that is a nagging pain.

There is a certain amount of discomfort that may accompany getting full mobility and strength back, but it's up to you to ensure that you're not mistaking injury-related pain for normal discomfort.

If you have a knee or ankle injury, be sure that you're careful when turning. Pushing off walls can aggravate certain conditions. If you have a leg injury, use a pull buoy.

As you can see, determining what caused your injury and what aggravates your injury not only will help you pick the best course of recovery but will decrease the likelihood that you will have the same injury later in life.

Injuries of the extremities can be extremely debilitating and, in most sporting platforms, be difficult to recover from because it's almost impossible to isolate the problem while keeping the rest of the body in shape. One of the most beneficial and unique advantages of swimming is that you can easily stay in shape while resting injuries.

While it's important to consult with your personal doctor on recovery from a serious injury, smaller problems can be fixed with a slow-paced training schedule that brings the injured area back into motion at an appropriate pace.

## CONDITIONING BY WATER RUNNING

All athletes require conditioning either to last through long bouts of physical activity or for repeats of short-term, intense activity. Athletes who have developed a strong core of conditioning through regular physical activity don't want to lose that if they become injured or otherwise cannot continue their training on land for a period of days, weeks, or even months.

Swimming the various strokes can be a great way to build and maintain physical endurance. As we've said time and time again, it's a full-body workout that can't be beat. But if you want some results in a hurry and don't want to work on your technique on certain days, or physically can't work out on land comfortably, you can still get fit or maintain fitness while being in the pool—and standing up. How? It's called "water running." And it's essentially done just the way it sounds.

The easiest way to get started in this is with the use of a deep-water running belt, which you put around your waist and it provides buoyancy for you. The most popular is called the AquaJogger. The best part about using these devices is that you have equal resistance all around your body. While wearing the belt, you simply simulate running in deep water. Professional football players are known to use this, as are triathletes.

Runners especially will love this form of exercise, but it enables more than rehabilitation. It's a great cross-training tool and a great conditioning method.

Depending on your goals, once you get in the water you'll be doing different things, but, as always, you want to make sure you take the time to warm up. When you're in the water, simply move around for a few minutes with easy sculling and easy kicking of the legs. If you'd prefer, you can warm up before you even put on the flotation device. That way, once you're in the belt and ready to go, you can just get started.

If you're looking for conditioning or recovery from an injury, make sure you start slowly. Don't tire yourself out too quickly; take strides just as you would on a track and put in varied amounts of time. It is necessary to mention that if you begin to feel any pain, you should stop right away.

Once you're comfortable with water running, slowly add more time. Before your heart rate can naturally be lower in the water than with the same activity on land, you'll want to add a few minutes to your workouts or increase the intensity just slightly. If you're in the water three days a week, try adding two to three minutes to your sessions every week until you find a period of time you're comfortable with.

For those not injured but taking advantage of this activity, take shorter strides and increase your intensity. Lifting the knees higher will also help increase your heart rate.

Be sure when doing this that you're not using your arms or leaning. Keep your hands loosely closed and, just as in running, let your feet do the moving for you. Kick the water behind you as you kick in running, and enjoy this simple but effective workout.

## SAMPLE REHAB PROGRAM

Many athletes develop stress fractures in their lower legs (in some cases their tibia, others their fibula) and feet (metatarsals). Generally these are highly competitive athletes who have had the misfortune of becoming injured during a part of their season that is generally high in mileage (for runners) or during intense drill work (basketball and many other sports) involving jumping, sprints, and so on. These athletes have a twofold problem. One, they are not only missing out on being able to keep training and developing their skills, but they're losing cardiovascular conditioning due to a lack of physical activity. Two, stress fractures generally can be solved (without surgery) only with rest. If the injury was caused by the sport itself, it makes sense that they can't simply go back to it and "shake it off."

Swimming, even for an athlete who has barely developed average skills in the water, can be a saving grace. As with most injuries, recovery should be self-paced. Below is an example of a healing program that allows for maintenance of the cardiovascular system and muscles while allowing rest for the affected body part. The outline is assuming an average or below-average proficiency in the pool.

Warm-up: Always warm up your entire body. Slow swimming, stretching (as described in other chapters of this book), water walking, and a slow increase in speed will help you avoid exacerbating an injury and will prevent new ones.

| Week | Workout | Notes |
|---|---|---|
| 1 (three days spread out evenly) | Water walking | Walk through the water lifting your knees high, moving through the water resistance. |
| 2 | Continued water walking | |
| 3 | All freestyle and backstroke pulling, maintaining a pace roughly 60% of your maximum capability.<br>Post warm-up, break your workout down with the goal of maintaining endurance.<br>For example:<br>Five sets of 200 yards continuous pulling (5 x 200) with 1 minute of rest between repetitions. | Make all of your turns "open turns," in that you're not flipping. Instead, touch with your hands, turn, and go. Do not push off the wall with your legs. If your injury is in only one leg, you may push gently with the injury-free leg.<br>Keep your volume of use appropriate for your level of fitness. Don't overdo it. |

Be sure you're not increasing your volume of use in the injured area too quickly. This is just an example of how to integrate your body into a swimming program slowly and build into recovery.

## UPPER-BODY INJURIES

For an upper-body injury, you have tools available to you that allow for immobilizing the arms in the water. If you have an injury of the biceps or triceps, forearms, or chest, you may find the use of a kickboard extremely useful. Both flutter kicking and breaststroke kicking are great ways to keep up your strength and get your heart rate up.

Keep in mind that if you have a shoulder injury, using a kickboard can do more harm than good. Because of your body angle, kicking with a board puts pressure on your shoulder joints. If your injury is isolated on one side, a better option is to kick without a board. For flutter kicking, move to your back and keep your injured arm at your side. Your other arm can extend toward the other end of the pool or also remain at your side. For breaststroke kicking, lead with the uninjured arm and have your injured limb down at your side.

In the case of a shoulder injury, also be sure you're not pulling yourself up on the wall with your hurt arm. These are the small things that often are neglected during swim rehab and can prevent a full recuperation.

## USING SWIMMING TO RECOVER FROM SWIMMING INJURIES

As in any form of physical activity, it is possible to become injured while swimming. The fortunate part, should this happen, is that it generally requires a simple fix. The leading causes of swimming injuries are inadequate preparation and inefficient technique.

If this should happen to you, go back to the basics. Evaluate your strokes and find what you're doing wrong. Once you've pinpointed these problems, make it your goal from that point on to rectify them. Not only will you be able to heal your injury, but you'll become a better swimmer at the same time.

While freak accidents can happen to anyone in any sport and cause the occasional problem, swimming injuries, while still fairly rare, generally occur in the rotator cuff and neck. Additional problems can occur in the groin from overuse, usually related to hard breaststroke kicking.

Problems in the neck are usually due to lifting the head and looking too forward, causing the neck to be at an odd angle both during the stroke and when you turn to breathe. Get back to keeping your head in the right line and maintaining that position when breathing, and you should soon find relief.

Problems in the shoulder and groin can be caused by overuse, but in the case of the former they can also occur from entering too far over your body when swimming. Be sure you're not overreaching, and also be sure you're not swimming without proper rotation, as this can cause unnecessary weight to be placed upon the shoulder.

All in all, if something is causing you pain, go back and review basic technique, and you should feel better soon.

# Final Thoughts

Well, you've read it all by now; the entire *Get Wet, Get Fit* program. Swim technique, sets, dryland training with and without weights, stretching, and nutrition, everything you need and then some. We've given you the tools, but, like construction equipment, they're useless unless picked up and put to work. We hope you'll take advantage of your new knowledge and use it to get into the best shape of your life. Your age or level of fitness doesn't matter right now, what's important is where you want to go and what you want to be.

Keep in mind these crucial dos and don'ts:

**Do** train hard in all you do: in the pool, in the gym, even in the kitchen.

**Don't** forget to stretch every single day. A little every day can go a long way.

**Do** drink enough water—for active people, at least a gallon throughout the day.

**Don't** smoke or use other harmful drugs. If you do, now is a great time to quit.

**Don't** be negative.

**Do** be positive. There's no limit to the benefits of mental health.

**Don't** quit. Whatever you do, don't give up on yourself. You're the only one who can accomplish your goals, and you're the only one who has the opinion that really matters. Be happy with yourself and you'll be happy with life.

## Olympian Tip Motivation

***Gary Hall Jr.—***
***ten-time medalist, 1996 Atlanta, 2000 Sydney, 2004 Athens Olympics***

To some extent I have thus far successfully managed my type 1 diabetes. I mean that as to say I haven't allowed diabetes to end my swimming career as some doctors told me it would. I have won six Olympic medals since being diagnosed. Perhaps more important, I don't have any of the terrible diabetes health complications. So many people turn to me for advice in how to deal with their various challenges.

I sometimes think of a great swimmer and friend of mine, Dean Hutchinson. While Dean wasn't short, he often appeared it when standing next to his competition.

Dean was a seven-time NCAA Division I All-American and U.S.A. National Team member. He was a cocaptain of Auburn's first-ever Southeastern Conference Championship team in 1994 and a flag bearer and silver medalist at the World University Games in 1999. Hutchinson's highest world ranking was eighth in the 50-meter freestyle in 1994. He competed in three Olympic Trials and captured Rookie of the Meet honors at the 1992 Olympic Trials.

Dean is currently a coach at Rider University.

While swimming, Dean had one of the best starts I have ever seen. Any height advantage that other swimmers had on Dean was negated by the time they had taken their first stroke.

He also had only one lung. In his own words, "It was June 29th, 1993, and I was 21. I had a very rare tumor that was causing seizures and I was coughing up a lot of blood. It actually happened at the NCAA Championships my sophomore year. Spit up blood on deck. They surgically removed the upper half of my left lung. It worked out pretty well in the end."

Ha! That gets me. "It worked out pretty well in the end." I love that, like, no big deal. I didn't die. Can you imagine looking over to the lane next to you and the guy is coughing up blood behind the blocks?

Lungs are pretty important in athletics, especially swimming, where you work as hard as any athlete in the world while holding your breath. But Dean didn't let losing a lung stop him from doing what he wanted to do.

So when you look at this guy and what he was able to do when most others would have used his obstacles as excuses, you realize that, barring some things that we don't have control over (obstacles come in many forms), we are ultimately, in the end, in control of our own destiny.

If you want to be a swimmer, be a swimmer. If you want something, really want something, obstacles like height, or diabetes, or even cancer can't stop you from pursuing it. If you are willing to work hard at it, you'll be amazed at what can't stop you.

Know what you want and go after it. First, take your time and decide what it is you want. It's great to have big goals, but know that it's small steps that take us to great places. It's going to take time and a lot of small steps.

There are going to be days that you feel like it can't be done because we all have days like that, but by identifying what you want and focusing on it you'll get through those days. Every swimmer goes through that. We ask ourselves questions like "Why am I doing this?" when things aren't fun.

It's a good question. Do you know the answer? There aren't any magic words that I can say that will make you leap from your bed every morning for the rest of your life exclaiming, "Today I will swim." because there are going to be days when you don't feel like getting out of bed. There are going to be days when you would rather be hanging out doing normal stuff with friends than at swimming practice. I will tell you that identifying what you like about swimming, why you are swimming, and focusing on that during those tough days will make getting through it a *lot* easier.

Motivation is an interesting thing. I believe that it comes from within. Either you are a motivated person who is willing to get the job done, no matter what, or you aren't. The motivated people are successful, people who change the world. The others walk away from a task when the going gets tough and drift from one thing to another. The "motivation" that we get from others is more like a reminder of something that we know deep down inside to be true, that we are in control of our own destiny. The right choices we make, coupled with some hard work, will take us where we want to go. Obstacles are just part of every person's life.

Standing on the blocks and racing feels great. Going a personal best time feels incredible. Why? You have accomplished something that you worked hard to achieve. It isn't something that you can buy or have someone do for you or give you. You have earned yourself self-respect, a sense of accomplishment, the good kind of pride, and confidence.

I guess that in some ways swimming teaches you a lot of valuable lessons about life that you probably won't even realize until you are much older. Words that are just words to others, like "commitment," "dedication," "goals," "hard work," "dreams," "ambition," and "motivation," take on new meaning when you have actually experienced what they are. Of course, it is your life and the decisions that you make are yours. Nobody makes all the right choices.

Are you motivated? It's a big choice because it's not just about making it to another swim practice. It's about making a life decision. Do you know what commitment is? Are you one day going to change the world? It's easier not to.

When you get to the top, though, all of those practices and aches and pains along the way seem worth it. As a matter of fact, you reflect on those struggles with fond memories. Know that it can be done. There are others out there who have faced worse and triumphed. If they can do it, you can, too.

Remember, champions are determined not by their victories but by how they deal with obstacles.

Dean Hutchinson never made the Olympic Swim Team. But that guy is an inspiration, a real champion who has made a difference.

What about you?

## Swimming Resources

By this point, you're a talented swimmer with the body to show for it and a newfound dedication to training and nutrition. You've made great strides to improve your life, we're very proud of you, and we hope you're proud of yourself as well.

If you've found a passion for swimming that just won't let up, you're not alone. It's an addictive adventure, and it's one that you can be a part of for a lifetime. If you want to know how to get involved in a formal program or just want to keep up with swimming or talk to other swimmers, below is a list of some resources you may find useful.

Official Page of USA Swimming—Club Information, Events: www.usswim.org

Official Page of FINA—International Governing Body: www.fina.org

United States Master Swimming—Resource for Swimmers 18 and Over, Forums: www.usms.org

Swimming Equipment—Suits, Goggles, Toys, and More: www.speedousa.com

Swimming Safety Tips: www.cdc.gov/healthyswimming/

Swimming News—Swimming News and Community: www.timedfinals.com

Swimming Radio—Swimming Audio Content, Forums: www.deckpass.com

Swimming Community—A "MySpace" for Swimmers and Fans: www.swimroom.com

College Swimming—News, Schedules, and Results: www.collegeswimming.com

Acknowledgments

We would like to express our most sincere gratitude to everyone who had a part in making this book possible, from its conception as a mere idea to the final product.

In no particular order we would like to thank:

Mollie Glick of the Jean V. Naggar Agency for finding this book a great home.

Amanda Patten and the team at Fireside for their faith in not just this project but this program.

All of the athletes and experts involved: Nick Brunelli, Rowdy Gaines, Scott Goldblatt, Gary Hall Jr., Tommy Hannan, Val and Joy Kalmikovs, Adam Mania, Russell Mark, Ed Moses, Gabe Woodward, and Dana Vollmer.

Our families: Don Anderson and Christena Warwick, Michael Jendrick, Tom and Janice Tani, Erin and Tom Quann, Laura Quann, and Michael Quann, and everyone else who offered early reviews and encouragement. And to a good friend who was a valuable assistant in research, Matt Nader.

# Index